CONGESTIVE HEART FAILURE Cookbook

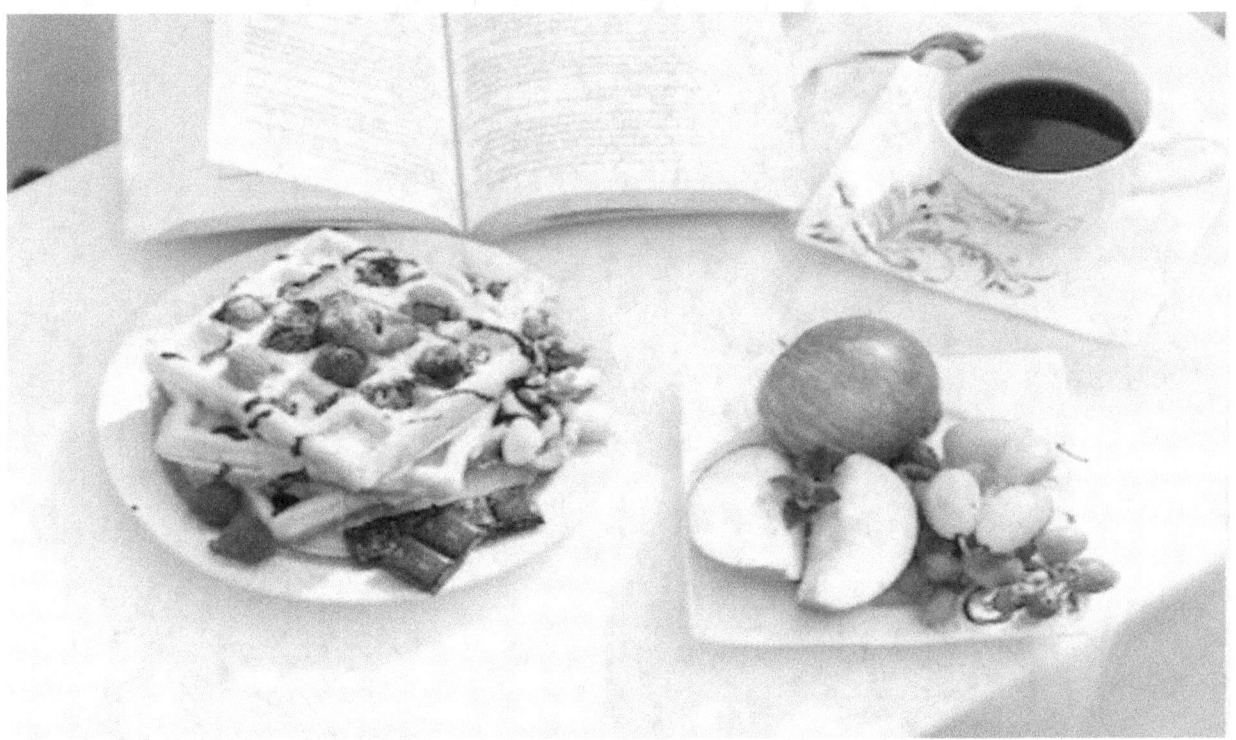

60 Essential Heart-Healthy Recipes & Lifestyle Tips for a Vibrant Life: 28-Day Meal Plan for Nourishment, Healing, and Hope

Monalisa Blake

Copyright©2024 Monalisa Blake

All Rights Reserved. No part of this publication may be reproduced, distributed, or transmitted in any form or by any means, including photocopying, recording, or other electronic or mechanical methods without prior written permission of the publisher, except in the case of brief quotations embodied in critical reviews and certain other noncommercial uses permitted by copyright.

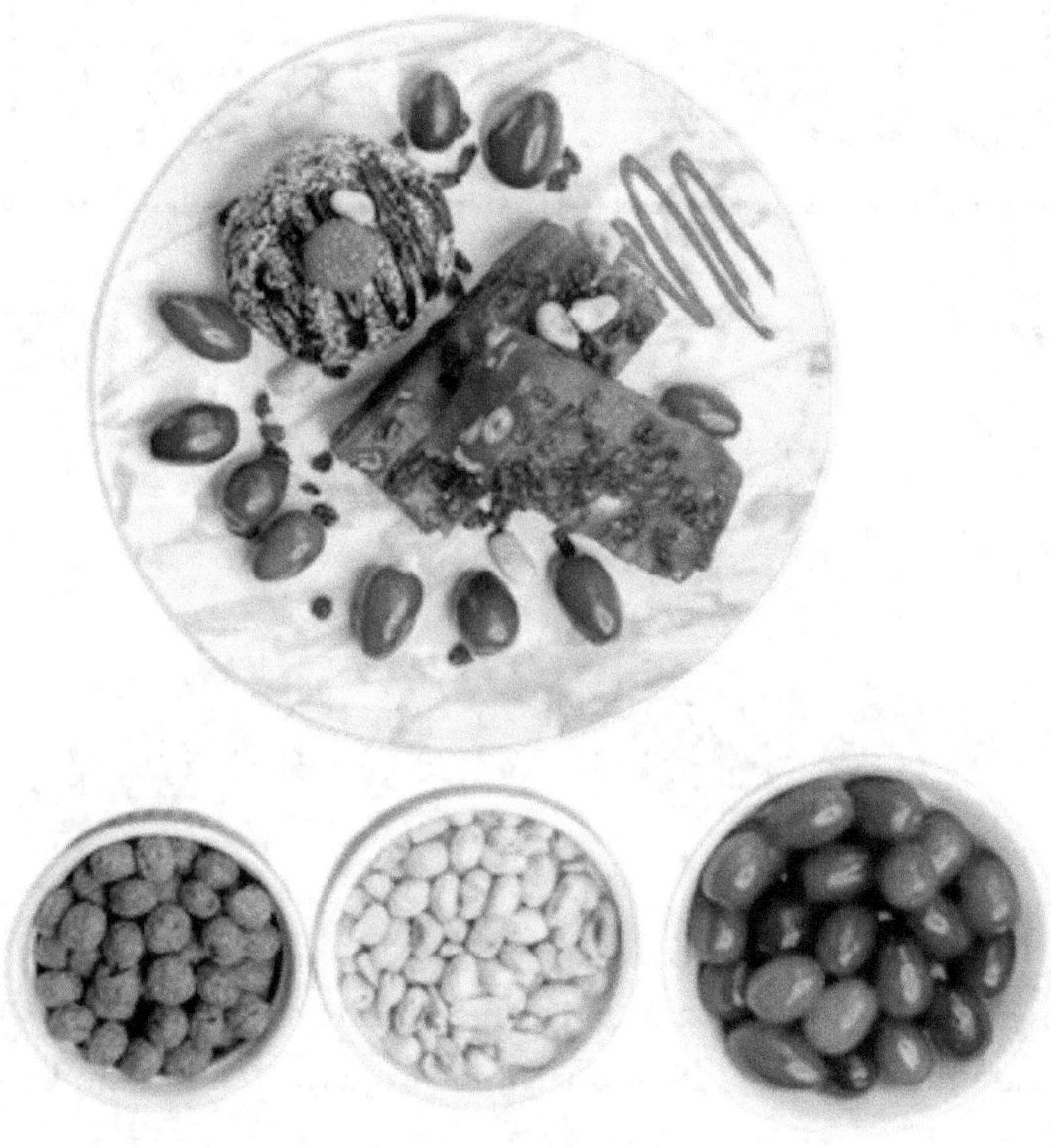

TABLE OF CONTENT

INTRODUCTION 7

- Understanding Congestive Heart Failure 9
- Understanding Congestive Heart Failure (CHF) 11
- Types of CHF 12
- Common Causes of CHF 12
- Common Symptoms of CHF 14
- Diagnosis and Treatment 15
- Living with CHF 16

CHAPTER 1: ESSENTIALS OF A HEART-HEALTHY DIET 17

- Practical Tips for Implementing These Guidelines: 20
- Importance of Balanced Nutrition for Congestive Heart Failure (CHF) 21
- Practical Tips for Achieving Balanced Nutrition: 23
- Key Nutrients for Heart Health 24
- Tips for Incorporating These Nutrients into Your Diet: 26
- Foods to Include and Avoid for Heart Health in Congestive Heart Failure (CHF) 27
- Meal Planning and Preparation for Congestive Heart Failure (CHF) 31
- Tips for Meal Planning and Grocery Shopping for Congestive Heart Failure (CHF) 34
- Preparing Your Kitchen for Heart-Healthy Cooking 38

CHAPTER 2: BREAKFAST RECIPES 41

- *Smoothie with Spinach and Berries* 41
- *Chia Seed Pudding* 42
- *Avocado Toast* 43
- *Greek Yogurt Parfait* 44

Oatmeal with Berries and Almonds 45

Quinoa Breakfast Bowl 46

Blueberry Buckwheat Pancakes 47

Spinach and Mushroom Egg White Omelette 48

CHAPTER 3: LUNCH RECIPES 49

Grilled Chicken Salad with Mixed Greens 49

Grilled Salmon with Asparagus 50

Lentil and Vegetable Soup 51

Turkey and Avocado Wrap 52

Quinoa and Black Bean Salad 53

Stuffed Bell Peppers with Brown Rice and Vegetables 54

Chicken and Quinoa Stir-Fry 55

Mediterranean Chickpea Salad 57

CHAPTER 4: DINNER RECIPES 59

Baked Cod with Asparagus and Lemon 59

Turkey and Vegetable Stir-Fry 60

Stuffed Bell Peppers with Quinoa and Black Beans 61

Roasted Chicken with Sweet Potatoes and Brussels Sprouts 62

Spinach and Ricotta Stuffed Shells 63

Slow Cooker Chicken Stew 65

Lentil and Vegetable Shepherd's Pie 66

Herb-Crusted Pork Tenderloin with Steamed Broccoli 67

CHAPTER 5: SNACKS AND APPETIZERS 69

Hummus with Veggie Sticks 69

Apple Slices with Almond Butter 70

Greek Yogurt with Honey and Walnuts 71

Spiced Chickpea Crunch 72

Baked Sweet Potato Chips 73

Caprese Skewers (Cherry Tomatoes, Basil, and Mozzarella) 74

Avocado and Black Bean Salsa.. 75

Cucumber and Tomato Salad... 76

CHAPTER 6: DESSERTS   77

Fresh Fruit Salad... 77

Berry Parfait with Greek Yogurt... 78

Chia Seed Pudding with Mango 79

Baked Apples with Cinnamon 80

Dark Chocolate-Dipped Strawberries 81

Oatmeal Raisin Cookies.. 82

Homemade Applesauce 83

Frozen Banana Bites with Almond Butter... 84

CHAPTER 7: SPECIAL DIETS AND MODIFICATIONS   85

Low-sodium options 85

Banana Oat Cookies... 85

Raspberry Lemon Sorbet 86

Poached Pears with Cinnamon 87

Pumpkin Spice Muffins.. 88

Almond Flour Brownies 89

Gluten-free alternatives 91

Baked Pears with Honey and Walnuts... 91

Chia Seed Pudding with Vanilla and Berries 92

Chocolate Avocado Mousse 93

Gluten-Free Lemon Bars 94

Mango Sticky Rice 95

VEGETARIAN AND VEGAN MODIFICATIONS 96

Raw Vegan Cheesecake 96

Vegan Pumpkin Pie 97

Vegan Chocolate Truffles 98

Vegan Lemon Poppy Seed Muffins 99

Vegan Peanut Butter Cups 100

DAIRY-FREE SUBSTITUTIONS 101

Vegan Chocolate Pudding 101

Coconut Milk Ice Cream 102

Date and Nut Energy Balls 103

Dairy-Free Apple Crisp 104

Avocado Lime Sorbet 105

CHAPTER 8: FITNESS AND LIFESTYLE TIPS   107

BENEFITS OF PHYSICAL ACTIVITY FOR CHF PATIENTS 111

GENTLE EXERCISES AND ROUTINES FOR CHF PATIENTS 113

TIPS FOR STAYING ACTIVE SAFELY WITH CHF 116

TECHNIQUES FOR RELAXATION AND MINDFULNESS 119

CHAPTER 9: 28-DAY MEAL PLAN FOR CONGESTIVE HEART FAILURE   123

WEEK 1 123

WEEK 2 125

WEEK 3 127

WEEK 4 129

CHAPTER 10: FREQUENTLY ASKED QUESTIONS   131

CONCLUSION 135

RECAP OF THE IMPORTANCE OF DIET AND LIFESTYLE IN MANAGING CHF 136

CONVERSION TABLE 139

VOLUME CONVERSIONS 139
WEIGHT CONVERSIONS 139
TEMPERATURE CONVERSIONS 140
COMMON INGREDIENT CONVERSIONS 140

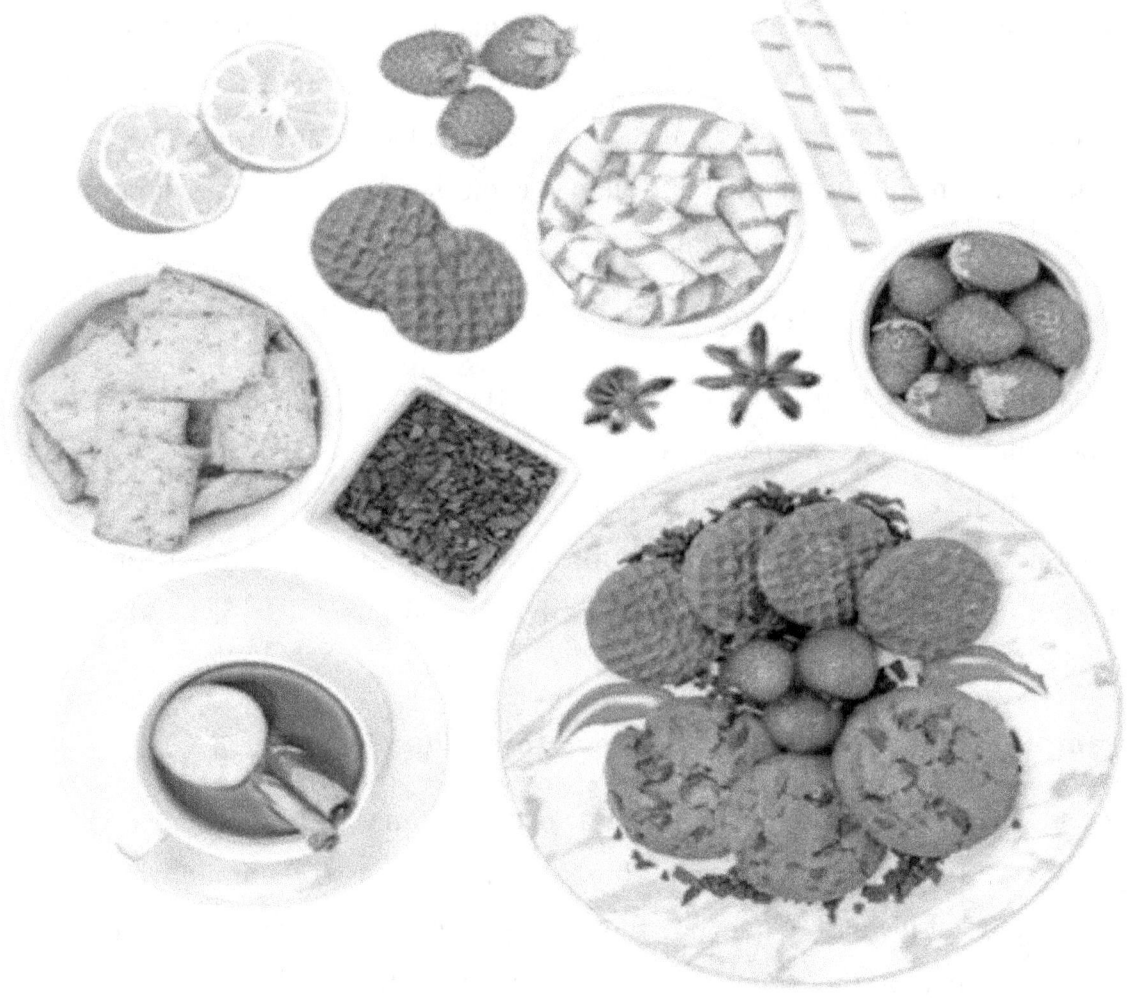

INTRODUCTION

Welcome to the **Congestive Heart Failure Cookbook**. This book is more than just a collection of recipes; it's a comprehensive guide designed to help you navigate the complexities of living with congestive heart failure (CHF) through the power of nutrition. Whether you're newly diagnosed, a caregiver, or someone looking to improve their heart health, this cookbook is crafted to support your journey towards a healthier, more fulfilling life.

The Importance of Diet in Managing CHF

Congestive heart failure is a chronic condition that affects millions of people worldwide. It can significantly impact your quality of life, but with the right lifestyle adjustments, you can manage your symptoms and improve your overall well-being. Diet plays a crucial role in this management. By making mindful food choices, you can reduce symptoms, prevent complications, and enhance your heart function.

Transforming Lives Through Nutrition

This cookbook aims to transform lives by offering practical, delicious, and heart-healthy recipes that cater to a variety of tastes and dietary needs. The recipes included are designed to be easy to prepare, nutritionally balanced, and packed with ingredients that support heart health. From energizing breakfasts to restorative dinners and guilt-free desserts, you'll find a wide range of options to keep your meals exciting and beneficial for your heart.

Championing Your Beliefs and Alleviating Your Fears

We understand that managing CHF can be overwhelming and that there are many fears and uncertainties associated with it. This cookbook is here to champion your beliefs in a better quality of life and to alleviate those fears by providing you with reliable, science-backed information and practical tips. Each recipe is thoughtfully created to help you make informed decisions about your diet, ensuring that you can enjoy your meals without compromising your health.

A Community of Support

You are not alone in this journey. This cookbook is a part of a larger community of individuals and caregivers dedicated to heart health. Throughout the book, you will find inspiring success stories, expert advice, and resources to help you stay motivated and informed. We encourage you to embrace this community and take charge of your heart health with confidence and optimism.

Our Commitment to You

As the author, my commitment is to provide you with the tools and knowledge you need to thrive despite the challenges of CHF. With over 17 cookbooks dedicated to health and nutrition, I have poured my expertise and passion into this book to ensure it meets your highest expectations. I believe that with the right guidance and determination, you can lead a vibrant and heart-healthy life.

Let's embark on this heart-healthy journey together. Here's to a future filled with delicious meals, better health, and a stronger heart.

Understanding Congestive Heart Failure

Congestive heart failure (CHF) is a chronic condition where the heart's ability to pump blood efficiently is impaired. This can lead to an accumulation of fluid in the lungs, liver, abdomen, and lower extremities, causing symptoms such as shortness of breath, fatigue, and swelling. CHF can result from various underlying conditions, including coronary artery disease, high blood pressure, and cardiomyopathy.

How CHF Affects the Body

In CHF, the heart's weakened pumping ability means that it cannot supply sufficient blood and oxygen to meet the body's needs. This inefficiency causes the following issues:

1. **Fluid Retention:** The kidneys may retain more fluid and salt, leading to swelling (edema) in the legs, ankles, and feet, as well as weight gain.

2. **Breathing Difficulties:** Fluid can accumulate in the lungs (pulmonary congestion), making it hard to breathe, especially during physical activity or when lying down.

3. **Fatigue and Weakness:** Reduced blood flow means muscles and tissues receive less oxygen, causing persistent tiredness and decreased ability to perform daily activities.

4. **Cognitive Impairment:** Poor blood circulation can affect brain function, leading to memory issues, confusion, and difficulty concentrating.

Impact on Daily Life

Living with CHF requires significant lifestyle adjustments to manage symptoms and prevent further heart damage. Here's how it can impact daily life:

1. **Dietary Changes:** A heart-healthy diet becomes crucial. This often means reducing sodium intake, limiting fluid consumption, and focusing on nutrient-rich foods to support heart health.

2. **Medication Management:** Patients typically need to take multiple medications, including diuretics, beta-blockers, and ACE inhibitors. Strict adherence to medication schedules is essential to control symptoms and improve heart function.

3. **Regular Monitoring:** Frequent monitoring of weight, blood pressure, and symptoms helps manage the condition and detect any worsening signs early.

4. **Physical Activity:** While exercise is beneficial, it must be balanced with rest. Activities are often modified to match the individual's capabilities, and overexertion should be avoided.

5. **Mental Health:** The emotional and psychological impact of living with CHF can be significant. Patients may experience anxiety, depression, or stress related to their condition and lifestyle changes.

6. **Social Life:** Fatigue and physical limitations can affect social interactions and participation in activities. Planning and pacing activities become essential to maintaining an active social life.

7. **Professional Life:** Work routines may need adjustments to accommodate fatigue and medical appointments. Some individuals might need to reduce hours or transition to less physically demanding roles.

Managing CHF

Effective management of CHF involves a multidisciplinary approach, including:

- **Medical Care:** Regular check-ups with healthcare providers to monitor heart function and adjust treatment plans.

- **Nutrition:** Adopting a diet that supports heart health and reduces fluid retention.

- **Exercise:** Engaging in safe, doctor-approved physical activities to strengthen the heart and improve overall fitness.

- **Education:** Learning about CHF and its management to make informed decisions and recognize early warning signs.

- **Support:** Accessing support from healthcare professionals, support groups, and loved ones to navigate the challenges of living with CHF.

By understanding CHF and its impact on daily life, individuals can take proactive steps to manage their condition and improve their quality of life. This cookbook aims to be a valuable resource in this journey, offering practical advice and delicious recipes to support a heart-healthy lifestyle.

Understanding Congestive Heart Failure (CHF)

What is Congestive Heart Failure?

Congestive heart failure (CHF) is a chronic progressive condition in which the heart muscle is unable to pump blood efficiently enough to meet the body's needs. This inefficiency can lead to a buildup of fluid in the lungs, liver, abdomen, and lower extremities. Unlike a heart attack, which is an acute event, CHF develops gradually over time as the heart becomes weaker.

How Does the Heart Work?

The heart is a muscular organ that pumps blood throughout the body. It has four chambers: two upper chambers called atria and two lower chambers called ventricles. Blood flows in a specific pattern:

1. Deoxygenated blood enters the right atrium, moves to the right ventricle, and is pumped to the lungs.

2. Oxygenated blood returns to the left atrium, moves to the left ventricle, and is then pumped out to the rest of the body.

In CHF, this cycle is disrupted, causing the heart to struggle in maintaining efficient blood flow.

Types of CHF

1. **Left-sided heart failure:** The left ventricle fails to efficiently pump oxygenated blood to the body. This can lead to fluid buildup in the lungs (pulmonary edema).
   - **Systolic failure:** The left ventricle loses its ability to contract normally.
   - **Diastolic failure:** The left ventricle loses its ability to relax normally because the muscle has become stiff.
2. **Right-sided heart failure:** The right ventricle fails to pump deoxygenated blood to the lungs. This can cause fluid retention in the lower extremities, abdomen, and other organs.
3. **Biventricular heart failure:** Both the left and right ventricles fail to pump blood adequately, combining symptoms of both left-sided and right-sided heart failure.

Common Causes of CHF

CHF results from various conditions that damage or overwork the heart muscle, leading to its weakening over time. Here are some of the primary causes:

1. **Coronary Artery Disease (CAD):**
   - The most common cause of CHF, CAD involves the narrowing or blockage of the coronary arteries, reducing blood flow to the heart muscle.
2. **High Blood Pressure (Hypertension):**
   - Chronic high blood pressure forces the heart to work harder, leading to thickening and stiffening of the heart muscle.
3. **Cardiomyopathy:**
   - Disease of the heart muscle itself, which can be inherited or caused by other factors such as infections, alcohol abuse, or drug use.

4. **Heart Valve Disease:**
    - Malfunctioning heart valves can disrupt blood flow through the heart, leading to CHF. Causes include congenital defects, infections, and aging.

5. **Arrhythmias:**
    - Irregular heart rhythms, such as atrial fibrillation, can cause the heart to beat too fast, too slow, or erratically, weakening the heart muscle over time.

6. **Congenital Heart Defects:**
    - Structural heart problems present from birth can impair the heart's ability to pump effectively, leading to CHF.

7. **Myocardial Infarction (Heart Attack):**
    - Damage to the heart muscle from a heart attack can significantly reduce the heart's pumping efficiency.

8. **Diabetes:**
    - Increases the risk of developing CHF due to associated high blood pressure, obesity, and damage to the heart muscle from high blood sugar levels.

9. **Chronic Kidney Disease:**
    - Kidney problems can lead to fluid and sodium retention, increasing blood pressure and putting additional strain on the heart.

10. **Sleep Apnea:**
    - This sleep disorder causes interrupted breathing during sleep, leading to low oxygen levels, increased blood pressure, and eventual heart strain.

11. **Lifestyle Factors:**
    - Smoking, excessive alcohol consumption, poor diet, and lack of physical activity contribute to conditions like hypertension, CAD, and obesity, increasing the risk of CHF.

Common Symptoms of CHF

Living with congestive heart failure (CHF) can be challenging due to its array of symptoms, which can vary in severity. Recognizing these symptoms early is crucial for effective management and improving quality of life. Here are the most common symptoms:

1. **Shortness of Breath (Dyspnea):**
    - Often occurs during physical activity or while lying flat.
    - May cause waking up feeling breathless at night (paroxysmal nocturnal dyspnea).

2. **Fatigue and Weakness:**
    - Persistent tiredness and a feeling of weakness, even during routine activities.

3. **Swelling (Edema):**
    - Swelling in the legs, ankles, feet, or abdomen due to fluid retention.
    - Can lead to sudden weight gain.

4. **Rapid or Irregular Heartbeat (Palpitations):**
    - Noticeable heartbeats, often described as fluttering or racing.

5. **Persistent Cough or Wheezing:**
    - A cough that produces white or pink blood-tinged mucus, often due to fluid buildup in the lungs.

6. **Increased Need to Urinate at Night (Nocturia):**
    - Frequent urination during the night as the body attempts to eliminate excess fluid.

7. **Swelling of the Abdomen (Ascites):**

- Accumulation of fluid in the abdomen, causing discomfort and bloating.

8. **Lack of Appetite and Nausea:**
   - Feeling full or experiencing nausea, which can lead to reduced food intake and weight loss.

9. **Difficulty Concentrating or Decreased Alertness:**
   - Cognitive issues such as memory problems, confusion, or difficulty focusing.

10. **Sudden Weight Gain:**
    - Rapid increase in weight due to fluid retention, often noticeable over a few days.

Diagnosis and Treatment

Diagnosing CHF involves a combination of medical history, physical examination, and diagnostic tests such as:

- **Echocardiogram:** Uses sound waves to create images of the heart, showing its size, structure, and motion.

- **Electrocardiogram (ECG):** Records the electrical activity of the heart to detect abnormalities.

- **Blood tests:** Measure levels of substances like B-type natriuretic peptide (BNP), which increase in heart failure.

- **Chest X-ray:** Shows the size and shape of the heart and lungs, detecting fluid buildup.

- **Stress test:** Evaluates heart function during physical exertion.

- **Cardiac MRI:** Provides detailed images of the heart's structure and function.

Treatment for CHF typically includes a combination of lifestyle changes, medications, and sometimes surgical interventions:

- **Lifestyle changes:** Dietary modifications, regular physical activity, smoking cessation, and weight management.

- **Medications:** Diuretics, ACE inhibitors, beta-blockers, and other drugs to manage symptoms and improve heart function.

- **Surgical treatments:** In some cases, procedures such as coronary artery bypass grafting, heart valve repair/replacement, or implantation of devices like pacemakers or defibrillators may be necessary.

Living with CHF

Managing CHF requires a comprehensive approach that includes medical treatment, lifestyle adjustments, and ongoing monitoring. By understanding the condition and adhering to a heart-healthy lifestyle, individuals with CHF can significantly improve their quality of life and reduce the risk of complications. This cookbook is designed to be a valuable resource, providing practical advice and delicious recipes to support a heart-healthy diet and overall well-being.

CHAPTER 1: ESSENTIALS OF A HEART-HEALTHY DIET

A well-balanced diet is crucial for managing congestive heart failure (CHF) and can help alleviate symptoms, reduce fluid retention, and enhance overall heart function. Here are the essential nutritional guidelines for individuals with CHF:

1. **Limit Sodium Intake**

    - **Why:** Sodium can cause fluid retention, exacerbating CHF symptoms such as swelling and shortness of breath.
    - **Recommendation:** Aim for less than 2,000 mg of sodium per day. Choose fresh, unprocessed foods and avoid adding salt to meals. Be cautious with canned, packaged, and restaurant foods, which often contain high levels of sodium.

2. **Monitor Fluid Intake**

    - **Why:** Excess fluid can lead to fluid retention and worsen CHF symptoms.
    - **Recommendation:** Follow your healthcare provider's advice on fluid limits, typically ranging from 1.5 to 2 liters per day. Include all fluids, such as beverages and soups. Use a daily fluid tracker to stay within recommended limits.

3. **Focus on Heart-Healthy Fats**

    - **Why:** Healthy fats can improve heart health by reducing inflammation and lowering cholesterol levels.
    - **Recommendation:** Incorporate sources of omega-3 fatty acids, such as fatty fish (salmon, mackerel), flaxseeds, and walnuts. Use unsaturated fats, like olive oil or avocado oil, instead of saturated and trans fats.

4. **Choose Whole Grains**
    - o **Why:** Whole grains provide essential nutrients and fiber, which help with digestion and overall cardiovascular health.
    - o **Recommendation:** Opt for whole grains like oats, quinoa, brown rice, and whole wheat products instead of refined grains. These can help regulate blood sugar and cholesterol levels.

5. **Increase Fruits and Vegetables**
    - o **Why:** Fruits and vegetables are rich in vitamins, minerals, and antioxidants, which support heart health and help manage blood pressure.
    - o **Recommendation:** Aim for a variety of colorful fruits and vegetables. Try to fill half of your plate with vegetables and fruits at each meal. Choose fresh or frozen options and limit those with added sugars or sodium.

6. **Manage Portion Sizes**
    - o **Why:** Controlling portion sizes helps in managing weight and reduces the strain on the heart.
    - o **Recommendation:** Use smaller plates and bowls to control portion sizes. Pay attention to serving sizes and avoid overeating, particularly with high-calorie or high-fat foods.

7. **Limit Processed and Sugary Foods**
    - o **Why:** Processed and sugary foods can contribute to high blood pressure, fluid retention, and weight gain.
    - o **Recommendation:** Reduce consumption of sugary snacks, desserts, and processed foods such as chips, cookies, and sugary drinks. Opt for healthier snacks like nuts, seeds, and fresh fruits.

8. **Ensure Adequate Protein Intake**
    - o **Why:** Protein is important for maintaining muscle mass and overall body function.
    - o **Recommendation:** Include lean protein sources like skinless poultry, fish, beans, lentils, and tofu. Balance protein intake to meet your needs without excessive consumption.

9. **Choose Low-Fat Dairy or Dairy Alternatives**
    - o **Why:** Low-fat dairy products or alternatives can provide necessary calcium and vitamin D without added saturated fat.
    - o **Recommendation:** Select low-fat or fat-free dairy options, or consider fortified plant-based alternatives such as almond milk or soy milk.

10. **Be Mindful of Potassium Levels**
    - o **Why:** Potassium helps balance fluid levels and control blood pressure but can interact with certain medications.
    - o **Recommendation:** Consult with your healthcare provider about your potassium needs. Include potassium-rich foods like bananas, oranges, and potatoes if appropriate for your condition and medication regimen.

11. **Incorporate Lean Proteins**
    - o **Why:** Lean proteins help maintain muscle mass and support overall health without adding excess fat.
    - o **Recommendation:** Choose skinless poultry, fish, beans, and legumes. Avoid fatty cuts of meat and limit red meat consumption.

12. **Monitor Blood Sugar Levels**
    - o **Why:** Managing blood sugar levels is important for overall health and can affect heart function.

- **Recommendation:** If you have diabetes or prediabetes, monitor blood sugar levels closely and choose foods with a low glycemic index.

Practical Tips for Implementing These Guidelines:

- **Plan Meals Ahead:** Prepare heart-healthy meals in advance to ensure adherence to dietary guidelines.

- **Read Labels:** Always check nutrition labels for sodium, fat, and sugar content.

- **Cook at Home:** Preparing meals at home allows you to control ingredients and avoid hidden sodium and unhealthy fats.

- **Stay Hydrated:** Drink water in moderation and follow fluid restrictions as advised by your healthcare provider.

- **Seek Professional Guidance:** Work with a registered dietitian or healthcare provider to tailor these guidelines to your individual needs and preferences.

Importance of Balanced Nutrition for Congestive Heart Failure (CHF)

Balanced nutrition is vital for managing congestive heart failure (CHF) and enhancing overall cardiovascular health. It ensures the body receives the necessary nutrients to function optimally, manage symptoms, and improve quality of life. Here's why balanced nutrition is crucial for individuals with CHF:

1. **Supports Heart Function**

   - **Why:** Balanced nutrition provides essential nutrients that help the heart pump blood effectively.

   - **Impact:** Adequate vitamins, minerals, and healthy fats support heart muscle function, regulate blood pressure, and manage cholesterol levels, which can help reduce the risk of complications.

2. **Manages Fluid Balance**

   - **Why:** Proper nutrition helps regulate fluid balance, which is crucial for managing CHF symptoms.

   - **Impact:** Limiting sodium and monitoring fluid intake can prevent fluid retention, reduce swelling, and alleviate symptoms such as shortness of breath and edema.

3. **Controls Blood Pressure**

   - **Why:** High blood pressure is a common cause of CHF and can exacerbate the condition.

   - **Impact:** A diet rich in potassium, magnesium, and fiber can help lower blood pressure. Consuming less sodium and incorporating healthy fats supports cardiovascular health and helps maintain healthy blood pressure levels.

4. **Aids in Weight Management**
    - o **Why:** Maintaining a healthy weight reduces the strain on the heart and can improve CHF symptoms.
    - o **Impact:** Balanced nutrition helps control calorie intake and promotes a healthy weight. Consuming a variety of nutrient-dense foods supports weight management while ensuring the body receives essential nutrients.

5. **Reduces Inflammation**
    - o **Why:** Chronic inflammation can worsen heart disease and CHF.
    - o **Impact:** A diet rich in antioxidants, omega-3 fatty acids, and anti-inflammatory foods helps reduce inflammation, improving overall heart health and potentially reducing the severity of CHF symptoms.

6. **Enhances Energy Levels**
    - o **Why:** CHF can lead to fatigue and reduced energy levels.
    - o **Impact:** A balanced diet provides the necessary energy and nutrients to support daily activities and overall well-being. A mix of carbohydrates, proteins, and healthy fats ensures sustained energy throughout the day.

7. **Supports Optimal Digestion**
    - o **Why:** Good digestion is important for nutrient absorption and overall health.
    - o **Impact:** A diet high in fiber from fruits, vegetables, and whole grains supports healthy digestion and prevents issues such as constipation, which can be problematic for those with CHF.

8. **Improves Overall Health**
    - o **Why:** A well-balanced diet contributes to overall health and well-being, impacting various body systems.

- **Impact:** Addressing nutritional needs supports other aspects of health, such as bone health, immune function, and mental well-being, which are integral to managing a chronic condition.

9. **Reduces the Risk of Complications**

    - **Why:** Proper nutrition can help prevent additional health issues that may arise with CHF.

    - **Impact:** A balanced diet can reduce the risk of developing related conditions such as diabetes, kidney disease, and other cardiovascular issues, thereby supporting long-term health and quality of life.

10. **Promotes Adherence to Treatment**

    - **Why:** Nutrition plays a role in the overall management of CHF, complementing medical treatments.

    - **Impact:** Following a balanced diet can enhance the effectiveness of prescribed medications and treatments. It helps manage symptoms, supports overall health, and may contribute to better outcomes.

Practical Tips for Achieving Balanced Nutrition:

- **Plan Balanced Meals:** Ensure meals include a mix of fruits, vegetables, whole grains, lean proteins, and healthy fats.

- **Read Nutrition Labels:** Pay attention to sodium, fat, and sugar content when selecting packaged foods.

- **Portion Control:** Manage portion sizes to avoid overeating and support weight management.

- **Stay Hydrated:** Follow fluid intake recommendations to manage CHF symptoms effectively.

- **Consult a Dietitian:** Work with a registered dietitian to develop a personalized nutrition plan tailored to your specific needs and health goals.

Key Nutrients for Heart Health

For managing congestive heart failure (CHF) and promoting overall cardiovascular health, focusing on key nutrients is essential. Each nutrient plays a specific role in supporting heart function, reducing risk factors, and maintaining overall well-being. Here are the key nutrients for heart health and their benefits:

1. **Omega-3 Fatty Acids**

    o **Why:** Omega-3 fatty acids help reduce inflammation, lower triglyceride levels, and improve heart rhythm.

    o **Sources:** Fatty fish (such as salmon, mackerel, sardines), flaxseeds, chia seeds, walnuts, and fortified foods.

2. **Potassium**

    o **Why:** Potassium helps balance fluid levels, supports proper muscle function, and helps control blood pressure.

    o **Sources:** Bananas, oranges, potatoes, spinach, tomatoes, and beans.

3. **Magnesium**

    o **Why:** Magnesium supports normal heart rhythm, helps regulate blood pressure, and contributes to muscle and nerve function.

    o **Sources:** Nuts, seeds, whole grains, leafy green vegetables, and legumes.

4. **Fiber**

    o **Why:** Fiber helps lower cholesterol levels, supports healthy digestion, and helps control blood sugar levels.

    o **Sources:** Whole grains, fruits, vegetables, legumes, and nuts.

5. **Antioxidants**

    o **Why:** Antioxidants help protect cells from damage caused by free radicals, reduce inflammation, and improve overall heart health.

- **Sources:** Berries (such as blueberries and strawberries), dark chocolate, nuts, green tea, and colorful fruits and vegetables.

6. **Vitamin D**
    - **Why:** Vitamin D supports heart health by regulating calcium levels and supporting overall cardiovascular function.
    - **Sources:** Fatty fish, fortified dairy products, egg yolks, and sunlight exposure.

7. **Calcium**
    - **Why:** Calcium is essential for maintaining strong bones and teeth, and it plays a role in muscle contraction and heart function.
    - **Sources:** Low-fat dairy products, fortified plant-based milks, leafy green vegetables, and almonds.

8. **Coenzyme Q10 (CoQ10)**
    - **Why:** CoQ10 is a powerful antioxidant that helps generate energy in cells and supports heart health.
    - **Sources:** Meat, fish, whole grains, and supplements.

9. **Vitamin B12**
    - **Why:** Vitamin B12 supports red blood cell formation and nerve function, which are crucial for heart health.
    - **Sources:** Animal products such as meat, poultry, fish, dairy, and fortified plant-based foods.

10. **Folate (Vitamin B9)**
    - **Why:** Folate helps reduce homocysteine levels, a risk factor for heart disease, and supports overall cardiovascular health.

- **Sources:** Leafy green vegetables, legumes, fortified cereals, and citrus fruits.

11. **Sodium**
    - **Why:** While sodium is essential in small amounts for fluid balance and nerve function, excessive sodium can contribute to fluid retention and worsen CHF symptoms.
    - **Sources:** Processed foods, canned soups, salty snacks, and table salt. (It is important to limit sodium intake in CHF management.)

Tips for Incorporating These Nutrients into Your Diet:

- **Eat a Variety of Foods:** Include a diverse range of nutrient-rich foods to ensure you get all the essential nutrients.

- **Choose Fresh and Whole Foods:** Opt for fresh fruits, vegetables, whole grains, lean proteins, and healthy fats.

- **Read Labels Carefully:** Be mindful of sodium, sugar, and fat content in packaged foods.

- **Cook at Home:** Preparing meals at home allows you to control ingredients and manage nutrient intake.

- **Consult a Dietitian:** Work with a registered dietitian to tailor your diet to your specific needs and health goals.

Foods to Include and Avoid for Heart Health in Congestive Heart Failure (CHF)

Managing congestive heart failure (CHF) involves making informed food choices to support heart health, control symptoms, and improve overall well-being. Here's a guide on which foods to include and avoid:

Foods to Include

1. **Fruits and Vegetables**

    o **Why:** Rich in vitamins, minerals, antioxidants, and fiber, they support heart health and help manage blood pressure.

    o **Examples:** Berries, apples, oranges, leafy greens (spinach, kale), carrots, broccoli, tomatoes.

2. **Whole Grains**

    o **Why:** Provide fiber, which helps lower cholesterol levels and stabilize blood sugar.

    o **Examples:** Brown rice, quinoa, oats, whole wheat bread, barley.

3. **Lean Proteins**

    o **Why:** Essential for maintaining muscle mass and overall health without adding excessive fat.

    o **Examples:** Skinless poultry, fish, tofu, legumes (beans, lentils), low-fat dairy.

4. **Healthy Fats**

    o **Why:** Support cardiovascular health by reducing inflammation and improving cholesterol levels.

    o **Examples:** Olive oil, avocado, nuts (walnuts, almonds), seeds (flaxseeds, chia seeds), fatty fish (salmon, mackerel).

5. **Low-Fat Dairy or Dairy Alternatives**
    - **Why:** Provides calcium and vitamin D without the added saturated fat.
    - **Examples:** Low-fat yogurt, skim milk, almond milk, soy milk.

6. **Foods Rich in Omega-3 Fatty Acids**
    - **Why:** Help reduce inflammation and lower triglyceride levels.
    - **Examples:** Fatty fish (salmon, sardines), flaxseeds, chia seeds, walnuts.

7. **Foods High in Potassium**
    - **Why:** Helps balance fluid levels and supports heart function.
    - **Examples:** Bananas, oranges, sweet potatoes, spinach, beans.

8. **Foods Rich in Magnesium**
    - **Why:** Supports normal heart rhythm and regulates blood pressure.
    - **Examples:** Nuts, seeds, whole grains, leafy green vegetables, legumes.

Foods to Avoid

1. **High-Sodium Foods**
    - **Why:** Excess sodium can cause fluid retention, worsening CHF symptoms.
    - **Examples:** Processed foods (canned soups, frozen meals), salty snacks (chips, pretzels), table salt, soy sauce.

2. **Saturated and Trans Fats**
    - **Why:** Increase bad cholesterol levels and contribute to heart disease.
    - **Examples:** Fatty cuts of meat, full-fat dairy products, margarine, commercially baked goods (cookies, pastries).

3. **Sugary Foods and Beverages**
    - **Why:** Can contribute to weight gain, high blood sugar, and increased risk of heart disease.
    - **Examples:** Sodas, sugary cereals, candy, desserts (cakes, pies).

4. **Refined Grains**
    - **Why:** Lack fiber and nutrients found in whole grains, and can contribute to blood sugar spikes.
    - **Examples:** White bread, white rice, sugary cereals, pastries.

5. **High-Cholesterol Foods**
    - **Why:** Can contribute to artery blockage and heart disease.
    - **Examples:** High-fat cuts of meat, fried foods, full-fat dairy products, shellfish (in high amounts).

6. **Processed and Packaged Foods**
    - **Why:** Often high in sodium, unhealthy fats, and added sugars.
    - **Examples:** Packaged snacks, instant noodles, ready-to-eat meals.

7. **Alcohol**
    - **Why:** Can contribute to fluid retention, increased blood pressure, and interact with medications.
    - **Examples:** Beer, wine, spirits. (If alcohol is consumed, do so in moderation and consult with a healthcare provider.)

8. **High-Sugar Snacks and Desserts**
    - **Why:** Can lead to weight gain and exacerbate heart-related issues.
    - **Examples:** Candy bars, cookies, cakes, ice cream.

Tips for Managing Food Choices:

- **Read Nutrition Labels:** Check for sodium, fat, and sugar content when purchasing packaged foods.

- **Cook at Home:** Preparing meals at home allows you to control ingredients and avoid hidden sodium and unhealthy fats.

- **Plan Balanced Meals:** Incorporate a variety of fruits, vegetables, whole grains, and lean proteins into your diet.

- **Use Herbs and Spices:** Flavor foods with herbs and spices instead of salt to reduce sodium intake.

Meal Planning and Preparation for Congestive Heart Failure (CHF)

Effective meal planning and preparation are crucial for managing congestive heart failure (CHF) and maintaining a heart-healthy diet. Here's a structured guide to help you plan and prepare meals that support your health:

1. Meal Planning

1.1. Set Goals

- **Why:** Establishing clear goals helps you focus your meal planning efforts and align with dietary needs.
- **Tips:** Set objectives for balanced meals, portion control, and adherence to CHF dietary guidelines. Aim for variety and nutritional adequacy.

1.2. Create a Weekly Menu

- **Why:** Planning meals for the week ensures variety and helps prevent unhealthy food choices.
- **Tips:** Plan for breakfast, lunch, dinner, and snacks. Include a mix of proteins, vegetables, whole grains, and healthy fats. Rotate recipes to maintain interest and balance.

1.3. Incorporate Heart-Healthy Foods

- **Why:** Ensures that meals adhere to dietary guidelines for CHF.
- **Tips:** Focus on fruits, vegetables, whole grains, lean proteins, and healthy fats. Avoid high-sodium, high-fat, and sugary foods.

1.4. Monitor Portion Sizes

- **Why:** Helps manage calorie intake and support weight management.
- **Tips:** Use measuring cups or a food scale to control portion sizes. Refer to dietary guidelines for recommended servings of different food groups.

1.5. Make a Shopping List

- **Why:** Ensures you purchase all necessary ingredients and reduces the risk of buying unhealthy options.
- **Tips:** Create a list based on your weekly menu, categorized by produce, proteins, grains, dairy, and pantry staples. Stick to the list to avoid impulse purchases.

2. Preparation and Cooking

2.1. Prep Ingredients in Advance

- **Why:** Saves time during the week and simplifies meal preparation.
- **Tips:** Wash, chop, and store vegetables and fruits. Cook grains, beans, or proteins in bulk and portion them for easy use throughout the week.

2.2. Practice Healthy Cooking Techniques

- **Why:** Retains nutrients and reduces the need for added fats or sodium.
- **Tips:** Opt for grilling, baking, steaming, or sautéing with minimal oil. Use herbs and spices for flavor instead of salt.

2.3. Prepare Balanced Meals

- **Why:** Ensures meals are nutrient-dense and aligned with CHF dietary guidelines.
- **Tips:** Include a lean protein source, whole grain, and a variety of vegetables. Incorporate healthy fats in moderation.

2.4. Use Portion Control

- **Why:** Helps manage portion sizes and prevent overeating.
- **Tips:** Serve meals on smaller plates to aid portion control. Use portion control containers for prepped meals.

2.5. Store and Reheat Properly

- **Why:** Ensures food safety and maintains meal quality.

- **Tips:** Store leftovers in airtight containers and refrigerate or freeze promptly. Reheat leftovers to the appropriate temperature.

2.6. Plan for Snacks

- **Why:** Helps manage hunger and maintain energy levels.
- **Tips:** Choose heart-healthy snacks like fresh fruits, vegetables with hummus, nuts, or yogurt. Portion snacks into individual servings.

2.7. Read Nutrition Labels

- **Why:** Helps make informed food choices and manage sodium, fat, and sugar intake.
- **Tips:** Check labels for sodium content and choose products with lower sodium. Be cautious with hidden sugars and unhealthy fats.

3. Practical Tips

3.1. Involve Family Members

- **Why:** Makes meal planning and preparation more enjoyable and considers everyone's dietary needs.
- **Tips:** Discuss dietary goals and preferences with family members. Involve them in meal planning and preparation.

3.2. Keep a Food Diary

- **Why:** Helps track dietary intake and identify areas for improvement.
- **Tips:** Record daily meals, snacks, and portion sizes. Note any symptoms or changes in health to discuss with your healthcare provider.

3.3. Adapt Recipes

- **Why:** Ensures recipes fit dietary needs and preferences.

- **Tips:** Modify recipes to reduce sodium, fat, and sugar. Experiment with herbs and spices for flavor without extra salt.

3.4. Seek Professional Guidance

- **Why:** Provides personalized advice and ensures dietary needs are met.
- **Tips:** Consult a registered dietitian to develop a personalized meal plan tailored to your specific health needs and goals.

Tips for Meal Planning and Grocery Shopping for Congestive Heart Failure (CHF)

Effective meal planning and grocery shopping are crucial for managing congestive heart failure (CHF) and adhering to a heart-healthy diet. Here's a structured guide to help you navigate these tasks:

1. Meal Planning Tips

1.1. Plan Weekly Menus

- **Why:** Provides structure and ensures balanced meals throughout the week.
- **Tips:** Plan meals for breakfast, lunch, dinner, and snacks. Include a variety of proteins, vegetables, whole grains, and healthy fats. Rotate recipes to keep meals interesting.

1.2. Set a Meal Planning Schedule

- **Why:** Helps maintain consistency and organization.
- **Tips:** Dedicate a specific day each week to plan meals and create a shopping list. Consider using a meal planning app or planner for convenience.

1.3. Focus on Heart-Healthy Ingredients

- **Why:** Ensures that meals adhere to CHF dietary guidelines.
- **Tips:** Incorporate plenty of fruits, vegetables, whole grains, lean proteins, and sources of healthy fats. Avoid high-sodium, high-fat, and sugary foods.

1.4. Prepare in Bulk

- **Why:** Saves time and effort throughout the week.
- **Tips:** Cook large batches of grains, beans, or proteins and portion them into individual servings. Store in airtight containers for easy access.

1.5. Utilize Leftovers

- **Why:** Reduces food waste and simplifies meal preparation.
- **Tips:** Plan meals that use leftovers creatively, such as turning roasted chicken into a salad or soup. Store leftovers properly and use them within a few days.

1.6. Create Balanced Meals

- **Why:** Ensures that each meal provides essential nutrients.
- **Tips:** Build meals around a lean protein source, whole grain, and a variety of vegetables. Include healthy fats in moderation.

1.7. Include Snacks in Your Plan

- **Why:** Helps manage hunger and maintain energy levels.
- **Tips:** Plan for heart-healthy snacks like fresh fruits, vegetables with hummus, nuts, or yogurt. Portion snacks into individual servings.

2. Grocery Shopping Tips

2.1. Make a Detailed Shopping List

- **Why:** Ensures you purchase all necessary ingredients and reduces impulse buying.
- **Tips:** Create a list based on your weekly menu, categorized by produce, proteins, grains, dairy, and pantry staples. Stick to the list to avoid unhealthy purchases.

2.2. Shop the Perimeter of the Store

- **Why:** Fresh produce, lean meats, and dairy products are often located around the store's perimeter.

- **Tips:** Focus on shopping the outer aisles for fresh fruits, vegetables, lean proteins, and dairy. Limit time spent in the inner aisles where processed and high-sodium foods are often found.

2.3. Choose Fresh and Seasonal Produce

- **Why:** Seasonal produce is often fresher, tastier, and more affordable.
- **Tips:** Select fruits and vegetables that are in season. Look for produce that is firm and free of blemishes.

2.4. Read Nutrition Labels Carefully

- **Why:** Helps make informed food choices and manage sodium, fat, and sugar intake.
- **Tips:** Check labels for sodium content and opt for products with lower sodium. Be cautious with hidden sugars and unhealthy fats.

2.5. Opt for Low-Sodium and Reduced-Fat Products

- **Why:** Supports heart health by reducing sodium and unhealthy fat intake.
- **Tips:** Choose low-sodium or no-salt-added versions of canned goods and processed foods. Select reduced-fat or fat-free dairy products.

2.6. Buy in Bulk When Appropriate

- **Why:** Can save money and reduce frequent trips to the store.
- **Tips:** Purchase non-perishable items like whole grains, beans, and spices in bulk. Ensure you have proper storage to keep these items fresh.

2.7. Be Cautious with Processed Foods

- **Why:** Processed foods can be high in sodium, unhealthy fats, and added sugars.
- **Tips:** Limit purchases of processed snacks, ready-to-eat meals, and canned foods with added salt. Opt for whole, unprocessed foods whenever possible.

2.8. Utilize Frozen and Canned Options

- **Why:** Provides convenience and can be cost-effective.
- **Tips:** Choose frozen fruits and vegetables without added sodium or sugar. Opt for low-sodium canned goods and rinse them before use if needed.

2.9. Practice Smart Shopping Habits

- **Why:** Helps manage budget and support a heart-healthy diet.
- **Tips:** Compare unit prices to get the best value. Use store flyers or apps for discounts on heart-healthy items.

2.10. Stay Hydrated

- **Why:** Proper hydration is essential for overall health, including managing CHF.
- **Tips:** Ensure you have a supply of water or low-sodium beverages on hand. Avoid purchasing sugary or high-sodium drinks.

Preparing Your Kitchen for Heart-Healthy Cooking

Creating a kitchen environment that supports heart-healthy cooking is essential for managing congestive heart failure (CHF) and adhering to a heart-healthy diet. Here's how to set up your kitchen for success:

Organize Your Pantry

Stock heart-healthy staples to ensure you have essential ingredients on hand. Include whole grains (such as brown rice and quinoa), low-sodium canned goods (like beans and tomatoes), healthy oils (like olive oil), and a variety of herbs and spices. Remove unhealthy items to reduce temptation and encourage healthier choices. Discard or donate high-sodium snacks, sugary foods, and processed items, replacing them with healthier alternatives. Use clear containers to keep track of pantry items and ensure freshness. Store grains, nuts, and spices in clear, airtight containers, and label them with contents and expiration dates.

Stock Your Refrigerator

Prioritize fresh produce, which is a key component of a heart-healthy diet. Keep a variety of fresh fruits and vegetables readily available, storing fruits in the crisper drawer and vegetables in perforated bags to maintain freshness. Choose lean proteins, such as skinless poultry, fish, and lean cuts of meat. Use the freezer for longer-term storage. Opt for low-fat dairy products, including milk, yogurt, and cheese, to support heart health by reducing saturated fat intake. Keep these items in designated areas of the refrigerator for easy access. Also, stock heart-healthy condiments like balsamic vinegar, low-sodium soy sauce, and natural mustard while avoiding high-sodium dressings and sauces.

Equip Your Kitchen

Invest in quality cookware to ensure you can prepare meals using healthy cooking methods. Non-stick or stainless steel cookware reduces the need for excessive oils, and appliances like a slow cooker or pressure cooker can add convenience. Equip your kitchen with essential tools, including measuring cups, spoons, a food scale, sharp knives, and cutting boards. A mandoline can be useful for uniform slicing of vegetables. Use proper storage containers to maintain food freshness and aid in portion control. Choose airtight containers for leftovers and prepped ingredients, and use portion control containers to manage serving sizes.

Maintain a Clean and Safe Kitchen

Practice proper food safety to prevent foodborne illnesses and ensure safe meal preparation. Wash hands, fruits, and vegetables thoroughly, and clean surfaces and utensils with hot, soapy water, especially after handling raw meat. Keep kitchen surfaces clean by wiping down countertops, stoves, and cutting boards regularly. Disinfect surfaces that come into contact with raw foods. Organize the refrigerator to maintain freshness and reduce cross-contamination. Store raw meats on the bottom shelf to prevent drips and keep ready-to-eat foods, like fruits and vegetables, on higher shelves.

Plan for Easy Cooking

Use meal prep techniques to streamline cooking and make meal preparation more manageable. Prepare ingredients in advance, such as chopping vegetables or cooking grains, and store prepped items in labeled containers for easy access. Label and date foods to ensure freshness and prevent food waste. Label containers with the date of preparation or freezing, use older items first, and regularly check for expired foods. Create a cooking routine to establish a consistent meal preparation process. Set aside specific days or times for meal prep to make cooking more efficient and less stressful.

CHAPTER 2: BREAKFAST RECIPES

Smoothie with Spinach and Berries

Prep Time: 5 minutes | **Cook Time**: 0 minutes | **Per Serving**: 1 serving

Ingredients:

- 1 cup fresh spinach leaves
- 1/2 cup mixed berries (strawberries, blueberries, raspberries)
- 1/2 banana
- 1 cup unsweetened almond milk
- 1 tablespoon chia seeds
- Ice cubes (optional)

Instructions:

1. Combine spinach, mixed berries, banana, almond milk, and chia seeds in a blender.
2. Blend until smooth and creamy.
3. Add ice cubes if desired and blend again.
4. Pour into a glass and enjoy the nutritious smoothie.

Nutritional Value (Approx.): Calories: 180 | Protein: 4g | Fiber: 7g | Healthy Fats: 5g | Carbohydrates: 30g

Chia Seed Pudding

Prep Time: 10 minutes | **Cook Time**: 0 minutes | **Per Serving**: 1 serving

Ingredients:

- 3 tablespoons chia seeds
- 1 cup unsweetened almond milk
- 1 tablespoon maple syrup or honey
- 1/2 teaspoon vanilla extract
- Fresh fruit for topping (optional)

Instructions:

1. In a bowl, combine chia seeds, almond milk, maple syrup, and vanilla extract.
2. Stir well to combine.
3. Let the mixture sit for about 10 minutes, then stir again to break up any clumps.
4. Cover and refrigerate for at least 2 hours or overnight until thickened.
5. Top with fresh fruit before serving if desired.

Nutritional Value (Approx.): Calories: 150 | Protein: 5g | Fiber: 10g | Healthy Fats: 7g | Carbohydrates: 14g

Avocado Toast

Prep Time: 5 minutes | **Cook Time**: 5 minutes | **Per Serving**: 1 serving

Ingredients:

- 1 slice whole grain bread
- 1/2 ripe avocado
- 1/2 lemon, juiced
- Salt and pepper to taste
- Red pepper flakes (optional)
- Cherry tomatoes, halved (optional)

Instructions:

1. Toast the slice of whole grain bread to your desired level of crispiness.
2. In a bowl, mash the avocado with lemon juice, salt, and pepper.
3. Spread the avocado mixture over the toasted bread.
4. Sprinkle with red pepper flakes and top with cherry tomatoes if desired.
5. Serve immediately and enjoy.

Nutritional Value (Approx.): Calories: 220 | Protein: 4g | Fiber: 9g | Healthy Fats: 15g | Carbohydrates: 20g

Greek Yogurt Parfait

Prep Time: 5 minutes | **Cook Time**: 0 minutes | **Per Serving**: 1 serving

Ingredients:

- 1 cup Greek yogurt (unsweetened)
- 1/2 cup mixed berries (strawberries, blueberries, raspberries)
- 1/4 cup granola
- 1 tablespoon honey or maple syrup
- 1 tablespoon chia seeds (optional)

Instructions:

1. In a glass or bowl, layer half of the Greek yogurt.
2. Add a layer of mixed berries and a sprinkle of granola.
3. Repeat with the remaining yogurt, berries, and granola.
4. Drizzle honey or maple syrup on top.
5. Sprinkle chia seeds on top if desired.
6. Serve immediately and enjoy.

Nutritional Value (Approx.): Calories: 250 | Protein: 15g | Fiber: 5g | Healthy Fats: 8g | Carbohydrates: 30g

Oatmeal with Berries and Almonds

Prep Time: 5 minutes | **Cook Time**: 10 minutes | **Per Serving**: 1 serving

Ingredients:

- 1/2 cup rolled oats
- 1 cup water or unsweetened almond milk
- 1/2 cup mixed berries (strawberries, blueberries, raspberries)
- 1 tablespoon sliced almonds
- 1 teaspoon honey or maple syrup (optional)
- Pinch of cinnamon (optional)

Instructions:

1. In a small pot, bring the water or almond milk to a boil.
2. Add the rolled oats, reduce heat to medium, and cook for about 5-7 minutes, stirring occasionally until thickened.
3. Remove from heat and let sit for a minute.
4. Top with mixed berries, sliced almonds, and a drizzle of honey or maple syrup if desired.
5. Sprinkle with cinnamon for added flavor.
6. Serve warm and enjoy.

Nutritional Value (Approx.): Calories: 220 | Protein: 6g | Fiber: 6g | Healthy Fats: 6g | Carbohydrates: 38g

Quinoa Breakfast Bowl

Prep Time: 10 minutes | **Cook Time**: 15 minutes | **Per Serving**: 1 serving

Ingredients:

- 1/2 cup cooked quinoa
- 1/4 cup unsweetened almond milk
- 1 tablespoon chia seeds
- 1/4 teaspoon vanilla extract
- 1/2 banana, sliced
- 1/4 cup fresh berries (blueberries, strawberries, raspberries)
- 1 tablespoon chopped nuts (almonds, walnuts, or pecans)
- 1 teaspoon honey or maple syrup (optional)

Instructions:

1. In a small pot, heat the cooked quinoa with almond milk over medium heat until warm.
2. Stir in the chia seeds and vanilla extract.
3. Transfer to a bowl and top with sliced banana, fresh berries, and chopped nuts.
4. Drizzle with honey or maple syrup if desired.
5. Serve warm and enjoy.

Nutritional Value (Approx.): Calories: 290 | Protein: 7g | Fiber: 7g | Healthy Fats: 10g | Carbohydrates: 42g

Blueberry Buckwheat Pancakes

Prep Time: 10 minutes | **Cook Time**: 10 minutes | **Per Serving**: 1 serving

Ingredients:

- 1/2 cup buckwheat flour
- 1/2 teaspoon baking powder
- 1/4 teaspoon baking soda
- 1/2 cup unsweetened almond milk
- 1 tablespoon maple syrup
- 1/2 teaspoon vanilla extract
- 1/4 cup fresh blueberries
- Coconut oil or cooking spray for the pan

Instructions:

1. In a mixing bowl, whisk together the buckwheat flour, baking powder, and baking soda.
2. Add the almond milk, maple syrup, and vanilla extract, and stir until combined.
3. Gently fold in the blueberries.
4. Heat a non-stick pan over medium heat and lightly grease with coconut oil or cooking spray.
5. Pour batter onto the pan to form small pancakes and cook until bubbles form on the surface, about 2-3 minutes.
6. Flip and cook for another 2-3 minutes until golden brown.
7. Serve warm with additional blueberries and maple syrup if desired.

Nutritional Value (Approx.): Calories: 200 | Protein: 5g | Fiber: 4g | Healthy Fats: 4g | Carbohydrates: 36g

Spinach and Mushroom Egg White Omelette

Prep Time: 5 minutes | **Cook Time:** 10 minutes | **Per Serving:** 1 serving

Ingredients:

- 3 egg whites
- 1/2 cup fresh spinach leaves
- 1/4 cup sliced mushrooms
- 1/4 small onion, diced
- Salt and pepper to taste
- Cooking spray or olive oil for the pan

Instructions:

1. Spray a non-stick pan with cooking spray or lightly coat with olive oil and heat over medium heat.
2. Add the diced onion and sliced mushrooms, cooking until soft, about 3-4 minutes.
3. Add the spinach and cook until wilted, about 1-2 minutes.
4. Pour the egg whites into the pan, ensuring they cover the vegetables evenly.
5. Cook until the egg whites are set, about 3-4 minutes.
6. Carefully fold the omelette in half and slide onto a plate.
7. Season with salt and pepper to taste.
8. Serve warm and enjoy.

Nutritional Value (Approx.): Calories: 90 | Protein: 12g | Fiber: 2g | Healthy Fats: 2g | Carbohydrates: 6g

CHAPTER 3: LUNCH RECIPES

Grilled Chicken Salad with Mixed Greens

Prep Time: 15 minutes | **Cook Time**: 10 minutes | **Per Serving**: 1 serving

Ingredients:

- 1 grilled chicken breast, sliced
- 2 cups mixed greens (lettuce, spinach, arugula)
- 1/2 cup cherry tomatoes, halved
- 1/4 cup cucumber, sliced
- 1/4 red bell pepper, sliced
- 1/4 avocado, sliced
- 2 tablespoons olive oil
- 1 tablespoon balsamic vinegar
- Salt and pepper to taste

Instructions:

1. In a large bowl, combine mixed greens, cherry tomatoes, cucumber, red bell pepper, and avocado.
2. Top with sliced grilled chicken breast.
3. In a small bowl, whisk together olive oil, balsamic vinegar, salt, and pepper.
4. Drizzle the dressing over the salad and toss gently to combine.
5. Serve immediately and enjoy.

Nutritional Value (Approx.): Calories: 320 | Protein: 30g | Fiber: 5g | Healthy Fats: 18g | Carbohydrates: 12g

Grilled Salmon with Asparagus

Prep Time: 10 minutes | **Cook Time**: 15 minutes | **Per Serving**: 1 serving

Ingredients:

- 1 salmon fillet (about 4 oz)
- 1/2 lb asparagus, trimmed
- 1 tablespoon olive oil
- 1 tablespoon lemon juice
- 1 clove garlic, minced
- Salt and pepper to taste
- Lemon wedges for serving

Instructions:

1. Preheat the grill to medium-high heat.
2. In a small bowl, combine olive oil, lemon juice, garlic, salt, and pepper.
3. Brush the salmon fillet and asparagus with the olive oil mixture.
4. Grill the salmon for 4-5 minutes on each side, until cooked through.
5. Grill the asparagus for about 5-7 minutes, turning occasionally, until tender.
6. Serve the grilled salmon with asparagus and lemon wedges.

Nutritional Value (Approx.): Calories: 300 | Protein: 28g | Fiber: 4g | Healthy Fats: 18g | Carbohydrates: 8g

Lentil and Vegetable Soup

Prep Time: 10 minutes | **Cook Time**: 40 minutes | **Per Serving**: 1 serving

Ingredients:

- 1/2 cup lentils, rinsed
- 1 small carrot, diced
- 1 celery stalk, diced
- 1/4 onion, diced
- 1 clove garlic, minced
- 1/2 cup diced tomatoes
- 2 cups low-sodium vegetable broth
- 1/2 teaspoon cumin
- 1/2 teaspoon paprika
- 1 bay leaf
- Salt and pepper to taste

Instructions:

1. In a large pot, sauté the onion, carrot, celery, and garlic over medium heat until softened, about 5 minutes.
2. Add the lentils, diced tomatoes, vegetable broth, cumin, paprika, bay leaf, salt, and pepper.
3. Bring to a boil, then reduce heat and simmer for 30-35 minutes, or until lentils are tender.
4. Remove the bay leaf before serving.
5. Serve hot and enjoy.

Nutritional Value (Approx.): Calories: 180 | Protein: 10g | Fiber: 12g | Healthy Fats: 2g | Carbohydrates: 34g

Turkey and Avocado Wrap

Prep Time: 10 minutes | **Cook Time**: 0 minutes | **Per Serving**: 1 serving

Ingredients:

- 1 whole wheat tortilla
- 3 slices deli turkey breast
- 1/4 avocado, sliced
- 1/4 cup shredded lettuce
- 1/4 cup sliced cucumber
- 1 tablespoon hummus
- Salt and pepper to taste

Instructions:

1. Lay the whole wheat tortilla flat and spread hummus evenly over one side.
2. Layer the turkey slices, avocado, shredded lettuce, and cucumber on top of the hummus.
3. Sprinkle with salt and pepper to taste.
4. Roll the tortilla tightly to form a wrap, securing with a toothpick if necessary.
5. Cut in half and serve immediately.

Nutritional Value (Approx.): Calories: 250 | Protein: 15g | Fiber: 6g | Healthy Fats: 12g | Carbohydrates: 24g

Quinoa and Black Bean Salad

Prep Time: 10 minutes | **Cook Time:** 15 minutes | **Per Serving:** 1 serving

Ingredients:

- 1/2 cup cooked quinoa
- 1/4 cup black beans, rinsed and drained
- 1/4 cup corn kernels
- 1/4 cup cherry tomatoes, halved
- 1/4 red bell pepper, diced
- 1 green onion, sliced
- 2 tablespoons fresh cilantro, chopped
- 1 tablespoon olive oil
- 1 tablespoon lime juice
- Salt and pepper to taste

Instructions:

1. In a large bowl, combine cooked quinoa, black beans, corn, cherry tomatoes, red bell pepper, green onion, and cilantro.
2. In a small bowl, whisk together olive oil, lime juice, salt, and pepper.
3. Pour the dressing over the salad and toss to combine.
4. Serve chilled or at room temperature and enjoy.

Nutritional Value (Approx.): Calories: 220 | Protein: 8g | Fiber: 7g | Healthy Fats: 8g | Carbohydrates: 32g

Stuffed Bell Peppers with Brown Rice and Vegetables

Prep Time: 15 minutes | **Cook Time**: 35 minutes | **Per Serving**: 1 serving

Ingredients:

- 1 large bell pepper, halved and seeds removed
- 1/2 cup cooked brown rice
- 1/4 cup diced tomatoes
- 1/4 cup black beans, rinsed and drained
- 1/4 cup corn kernels
- 1/4 cup diced zucchini
- 1 tablespoon olive oil
- 1/2 teaspoon cumin
- 1/2 teaspoon paprika
- Salt and pepper to taste

Instructions:

1. Preheat the oven to 375°F (190°C).
2. In a large bowl, combine cooked brown rice, diced tomatoes, black beans, corn, zucchini, olive oil, cumin, paprika, salt, and pepper.
3. Stuff each bell pepper half with the rice and vegetable mixture.
4. Place stuffed peppers in a baking dish and cover with foil.
5. Bake for 30 minutes, then remove foil and bake for an additional 5 minutes until peppers are tender.
6. Serve warm and enjoy.

Nutritional Value (Approx.): Calories: 250 | Protein: 6g | Fiber: 8g | Healthy Fats: 7g | Carbohydrates: 42g

Chicken and Quinoa Stir-Fry

Prep Time: 10 minutes | **Cook Time**: 20 minutes | **Per Serving**: 1 serving

Ingredients:

- 1/2 cup cooked quinoa
- 1 chicken breast, diced
- 1/2 cup broccoli florets
- 1/2 red bell pepper, sliced
- 1/4 cup sliced carrots
- 1/4 cup snap peas
- 1 tablespoon olive oil
- 1 clove garlic, minced
- 1 tablespoon low-sodium soy sauce
- 1 tablespoon sesame oil
- Salt and pepper to taste

Instructions:

1. In a large pan, heat olive oil over medium-high heat.
2. Add diced chicken breast and cook until browned and cooked through, about 5-7 minutes.
3. Add garlic, broccoli, red bell pepper, carrots, and snap peas, and cook for another 5 minutes until vegetables are tender.

4. Stir in cooked quinoa, soy sauce, sesame oil, salt, and pepper.

5. Cook for an additional 3 minutes, stirring frequently.

6. Serve warm and enjoy.

Nutritional Value (Approx.): Calories: 350 | Protein: 30g | Fiber: 6g | Healthy Fats: 14g | Carbohydrates: 28g

Mediterranean Chickpea Salad

Prep Time: 10 minutes | **Cook Time:** 0 minutes | **Per Serving:** 1 serving

Ingredients:

- 1 cup chickpeas, rinsed and drained
- 1/2 cup cherry tomatoes, halved
- 1/4 cup cucumber, diced
- 1/4 cup red onion, diced
- 1/4 cup Kalamata olives, sliced
- 2 tablespoons crumbled feta cheese
- 2 tablespoons olive oil
- 1 tablespoon lemon juice
- 1 teaspoon dried oregano
- Salt and pepper to taste

Instructions:

1. In a large bowl, combine chickpeas, cherry tomatoes, cucumber, red onion, and Kalamata olives.
2. In a small bowl, whisk together olive oil, lemon juice, oregano, salt, and pepper.
3. Pour the dressing over the chickpea mixture and toss to combine.
4. Sprinkle with crumbled feta cheese.
5. Serve immediately or refrigerate until ready to serve.

Nutritional Value (Approx.): Calories: 320 | Protein: 10g | Fiber: 8g | Healthy Fats: 22g | Carbohydrates: 26g

CHAPTER 4: DINNER RECIPES

Baked Cod with Asparagus and Lemon

Prep Time: 10 minutes | **Cook Time**: 20 minutes | **Per Serving**: 1 serving

Ingredients:

- 1 cod fillet (about 4 oz)
- 1/2 lb asparagus, trimmed
- 1 tablespoon olive oil
- 1 lemon, sliced
- 1 clove garlic, minced
- Salt and pepper to taste

Instructions:

1. Preheat the oven to 400°F (200°C).
2. Place the cod fillet and asparagus on a baking sheet.
3. Drizzle with olive oil and sprinkle with minced garlic, salt, and pepper.
4. Arrange lemon slices over the cod and asparagus.
5. Bake for 15-20 minutes, until the cod is cooked through and the asparagus is tender.
6. Serve warm and enjoy.

Nutritional Value (Approx.): Calories: 250 | Protein: 25g | Fiber: 4g | Healthy Fats: 12g | Carbohydrates: 10g

Turkey and Vegetable Stir-Fry

Prep Time: 10 minutes | **Cook Time**: 15 minutes | **Per Serving**: 1 serving

Ingredients:

- 1/2 lb ground turkey
- 1/2 cup broccoli florets
- 1/2 red bell pepper, sliced
- 1/4 cup sliced carrots
- 1/4 cup snap peas
- 1 tablespoon olive oil
- 1 clove garlic, minced
- 1 tablespoon low-sodium soy sauce
- 1 tablespoon sesame oil
- Salt and pepper to taste

Instructions:

1. In a large pan, heat olive oil over medium-high heat.
2. Add ground turkey and cook until browned and cooked through, about 5-7 minutes.
3. Add garlic, broccoli, red bell pepper, carrots, and snap peas, and cook for another 5 minutes until vegetables are tender.
4. Stir in soy sauce, sesame oil, salt, and pepper.
5. Cook for an additional 3 minutes, stirring frequently.
6. Serve warm and enjoy.

Nutritional Value (Approx.): Calories: 300 | Protein: 28g | Fiber: 5g | Healthy Fats: 18g | Carbohydrates: 10g

Stuffed Bell Peppers with Quinoa and Black Beans

Prep Time: 15 minutes | **Cook Time**: 35 minutes | **Per Serving**: 1 serving

Ingredients:

- 1 large bell pepper, halved and seeds removed
- 1/2 cup cooked quinoa
- 1/4 cup black beans, rinsed and drained
- 1/4 cup diced tomatoes
- 1/4 cup corn kernels
- 1/4 cup diced zucchini
- 1 tablespoon olive oil
- 1/2 teaspoon cumin
- 1/2 teaspoon paprika
- Salt and pepper to taste

Instructions:

1. Preheat the oven to 375°F (190°C).
2. In a large bowl, combine cooked quinoa, black beans, diced tomatoes, corn, zucchini, olive oil, cumin, paprika, salt, and pepper.
3. Stuff each bell pepper half with the quinoa and vegetable mixture.
4. Place stuffed peppers in a baking dish and cover with foil.

5. Bake for 30 minutes, then remove foil and bake for an additional 5 minutes until peppers are tender.

6. Serve warm and enjoy.

Nutritional Value (Approx.): Calories: 250 | Protein: 7g | Fiber: 8g | Healthy Fats: 8g | Carbohydrates: 42g

Roasted Chicken with Sweet Potatoes and Brussels Sprouts

Prep Time: 10 minutes | **Cook Time**: 40 minutes | **Per Serving**: 1 serving

Ingredients:

- 1 chicken breast, bone-in and skin-on
- 1 medium sweet potato, peeled and cubed
- 1 cup Brussels sprouts, halved
- 2 tablespoons olive oil
- 1 teaspoon dried thyme
- 1 teaspoon dried rosemary
- Salt and pepper to taste

Instructions:

1. Preheat the oven to 400°F (200°C).

2. In a large bowl, toss sweet potatoes and Brussels sprouts with olive oil, thyme, rosemary, salt, and pepper.

3. Place the chicken breast on a baking sheet and arrange the sweet potatoes and Brussels sprouts around it.

4. Roast for 35-40 minutes, until the chicken is cooked through and the vegetables are tender.

5. Serve warm and enjoy.

Nutritional Value (Approx.): Calories: 400 | Protein: 35g | Fiber: 8g | Healthy Fats: 20g | Carbohydrates: 28g

Spinach and Ricotta Stuffed Shells

Prep Time: 20 minutes | **Cook Time**: 30 minutes | **Per Serving**: 1 serving

Ingredients:

- 6 jumbo pasta shells
- 1/2 cup ricotta cheese
- 1/2 cup spinach, chopped
- 1 clove garlic, minced
- 1/4 cup grated Parmesan cheese
- 1/2 cup marinara sauce
- 1 tablespoon olive oil
- Salt and pepper to taste

Instructions:

1. Preheat the oven to 375°F (190°C).
2. Cook the pasta shells according to package instructions. Drain and set aside.
3. In a bowl, combine ricotta cheese, spinach, garlic, Parmesan cheese, salt, and pepper.
4. Stuff each shell with the ricotta mixture.

5. Spread half of the marinara sauce on the bottom of a baking dish. Arrange stuffed shells on top.

6. Drizzle the remaining marinara sauce over the shells.

7. Cover with foil and bake for 20 minutes. Remove foil and bake for an additional 10 minutes.

8. Serve warm and enjoy.

Nutritional Value (Approx.): Calories: 300 | Protein: 14g | Fiber: 4g | Healthy Fats: 12g | Carbohydrates: 34g

Slow Cooker Chicken Stew

Prep Time: 15 minutes | **Cook Time**: 6 hours | **Per Serving**: 1 serving

Ingredients:

- 1 chicken breast, diced
- 1 small carrot, sliced
- 1 celery stalk, sliced
- 1/2 cup diced potatoes
- 1/4 cup frozen peas
- 1/2 onion, diced
- 2 cups low-sodium chicken broth
- 1 tablespoon olive oil
- 1 teaspoon dried thyme
- 1 bay leaf
- Salt and pepper to taste

Instructions:

1. In a slow cooker, combine diced chicken, carrot, celery, potatoes, peas, and onion.
2. Add chicken broth, olive oil, thyme, bay leaf, salt, and pepper.
3. Cover and cook on low for 6 hours, or until vegetables are tender and chicken is cooked through.
4. Remove the bay leaf before serving.
5. Serve hot and enjoy.

Nutritional Value (Approx.): Calories: 250 | Protein: 25g | Fiber: 4g | Healthy Fats: 8g | Carbohydrates: 22g

Lentil and Vegetable Shepherd's Pie

Prep Time: 20 minutes | **Cook Time**: 30 minutes | **Per Serving**: 1 serving

Ingredients:

- 1/2 cup cooked lentils
- 1/2 cup diced carrots
- 1/2 cup peas
- 1/2 cup corn kernels
- 1/4 cup diced onion
- 1 clove garlic, minced
- 1 cup mashed potatoes
- 1 tablespoon olive oil
- 1 teaspoon dried thyme
- Salt and pepper to taste

Instructions:

1. Preheat the oven to 375°F (190°C).
2. In a pan, heat olive oil over medium heat. Add onion and garlic, and sauté until softened.
3. Add carrots, peas, corn, lentils, thyme, salt, and pepper. Cook for 5 minutes, stirring occasionally.
4. Transfer the vegetable mixture to a baking dish and spread evenly.
5. Top with mashed potatoes, spreading them evenly over the vegetables.
6. Bake for 25-30 minutes, until the top is golden brown.
7. Serve warm and enjoy.

Nutritional Value (Approx.): Calories: 300 | Protein: 10g | Fiber: 8g | Healthy Fats: 10g | Carbohydrates: 45g

Herb-Crusted Pork Tenderloin with Steamed Broccoli

Prep Time: 10 minutes | **Cook Time:** 25 minutes | **Per Serving:** 1 serving

Ingredients:

- 1 pork tenderloin (about 4 oz)
- 1 cup broccoli florets
- 1 tablespoon olive oil
- 1 clove garlic, minced
- 1 teaspoon dried rosemary
- 1 teaspoon dried thyme
- Salt and pepper to taste

Instructions:

1. Preheat the oven to 400°F (200°C).
2. In a small bowl, combine olive oil, garlic, rosemary, thyme, salt, and pepper.
3. Rub the mixture over the pork tenderloin.
4. Place the tenderloin on a baking sheet and roast for 20-25 minutes, until the internal temperature reaches 145°F (63°C).
5. While the pork is roasting, steam the broccoli until tender, about 5-7 minutes.
6. Serve the herb-crusted pork tenderloin with steamed broccoli.

Nutritional Value (Approx.): Calories: 280 | Protein: 28g | Fiber: 4g | Healthy Fats: 14g | Carbohydrates: 8g

CHAPTER 5: SNACKS AND APPETIZERS

Hummus with Veggie Sticks

Prep Time: 10 minutes | **Cook Time**: 0 minutes | **Per Serving**: 1 serving

Ingredients:

- 1/2 cup hummus
- 1 carrot, cut into sticks
- 1 celery stalk, cut into sticks
- 1/2 red bell pepper, sliced
- 1/2 cucumber, sliced

Instructions:

1. Arrange the carrot sticks, celery sticks, red bell pepper slices, and cucumber slices on a plate.
2. Serve with hummus on the side for dipping.
3. Enjoy this quick and nutritious snack.

Nutritional Value (Approx.): Calories: 180 | Protein: 6g | Fiber: 7g | Healthy Fats: 8g | Carbohydrates: 22g

Apple Slices with Almond Butter

Prep Time: 5 minutes | **Cook Time**: 0 minutes | **Per Serving**: 1 serving

Ingredients:

- 1 apple, cored and sliced
- 2 tablespoons almond butter

Instructions:

1. Arrange the apple slices on a plate.
2. Serve with almond butter on the side for dipping.
3. Enjoy this simple and satisfying snack.

Nutritional Value (Approx.): Calories: 250 | Protein: 4g | Fiber: 6g | Healthy Fats: 16g | Carbohydrates: 25g

Greek Yogurt with Honey and Walnuts

Prep Time: 5 minutes | **Cook Time:** 0 minutes | **Per Serving:** 1 serving

Ingredients:

- 1 cup plain Greek yogurt
- 1 tablespoon honey
- 2 tablespoons chopped walnuts

Instructions:

1. Spoon the Greek yogurt into a bowl.
2. Drizzle honey over the yogurt.
3. Sprinkle chopped walnuts on top.
4. Enjoy this delicious and nutritious snack.

Nutritional Value (Approx.): Calories: 280 | Protein: 15g | Fiber: 2g | Healthy Fats: 14g | Carbohydrates: 25g

Spiced Chickpea Crunch

Prep Time: 5 minutes | **Cook Time:** 25 minutes | **Per Serving:** 1 serving

Ingredients:

- 1 cup canned chickpeas, rinsed and drained
- 1 tablespoon olive oil
- 1/2 teaspoon smoked paprika
- 1/2 teaspoon cumin
- 1/4 teaspoon garlic powder
- Salt to taste

Instructions:

1. Preheat the oven to 400°F (200°C).
2. Pat the chickpeas dry with a paper towel.
3. In a bowl, toss the chickpeas with olive oil, smoked paprika, cumin, garlic powder, and salt.
4. Spread the chickpeas on a baking sheet in a single layer.
5. Bake for 20-25 minutes, shaking the pan halfway through, until the chickpeas are crispy.
6. Allow to cool slightly before serving.
7. Enjoy this crunchy and flavorful snack.

Nutritional Value (Approx.): Calories: 200 | Protein: 7g | Fiber: 6g | Healthy Fats: 10g | Carbohydrates: 22g

Baked Sweet Potato Chips

Prep Time: 10 minutes | **Cook Time**: 25 minutes | **Per Serving**: 1 serving

Ingredients:

- 1 medium sweet potato, thinly sliced
- 1 tablespoon olive oil
- 1/2 teaspoon sea salt
- 1/4 teaspoon paprika

Instructions:

1. Preheat the oven to 400°F (200°C).
2. In a bowl, toss the sweet potato slices with olive oil, sea salt, and paprika.
3. Arrange the slices in a single layer on a baking sheet lined with parchment paper.
4. Bake for 20-25 minutes, flipping halfway through, until crispy and golden.
5. Allow to cool slightly before serving.
6. Enjoy this healthy and crunchy snack.

Nutritional Value (Approx.): Calories: 150 | Protein: 2g | Fiber: 4g | Healthy Fats: 7g | Carbohydrates: 22g

Caprese Skewers (Cherry Tomatoes, Basil, and Mozzarella)

Prep Time: 10 minutes | **Cook Time**: 0 minutes | **Per Serving**: 1 serving

Ingredients:

- 10 cherry tomatoes
- 10 fresh basil leaves
- 10 small mozzarella balls (bocconcini)
- 1 tablespoon balsamic glaze (optional)

Instructions:

1. On each skewer, thread one cherry tomato, one basil leaf, and one mozzarella ball.
2. Arrange the skewers on a serving plate.
3. Drizzle with balsamic glaze if desired.
4. Enjoy this refreshing and easy-to-make snack.

Nutritional Value (Approx.): Calories: 200 | Protein: 10g | Fiber: 2g | Healthy Fats: 12g | Carbohydrates: 8g

Avocado and Black Bean Salsa

Prep Time: 10 minutes | **Cook Time:** 0 minutes | **Per Serving:** 1 serving

Ingredients:

- 1 ripe avocado, diced
- 1/2 cup black beans, rinsed and drained
- 1/2 cup cherry tomatoes, quartered
- 1/4 cup red onion, finely diced
- 1 tablespoon lime juice
- 1 tablespoon cilantro, chopped
- Salt and pepper to taste

Instructions:

1. In a bowl, combine avocado, black beans, cherry tomatoes, red onion, lime juice, cilantro, salt, and pepper.
2. Gently toss to mix the ingredients.
3. Serve immediately or chill for 10 minutes for flavors to meld.
4. Enjoy this delicious and nutritious snack.

Nutritional Value (Approx.): Calories: 220 | Protein: 5g | Fiber: 10g | Healthy Fats: 14g | Carbohydrates: 20g

Cucumber and Tomato Salad

Prep Time: 10 minutes | **Cook Time:** 0 minutes | **Per Serving:** 1 serving

Ingredients:

- 1 cucumber, sliced
- 1 cup cherry tomatoes, halved
- 1/4 cup red onion, thinly sliced
- 2 tablespoons olive oil
- 1 tablespoon red wine vinegar
- 1 teaspoon dried oregano
- Salt and pepper to taste

Instructions:

1. In a large bowl, combine cucumber slices, cherry tomato halves, and red onion slices.
2. In a small bowl, whisk together olive oil, red wine vinegar, dried oregano, salt, and pepper.
3. Pour the dressing over the vegetables and toss to coat.
4. Serve immediately or refrigerate for 15 minutes for flavors to develop.
5. Enjoy this light and refreshing salad.

Nutritional Value (Approx.): Calories: 150 | Protein: 2g | Fiber: 3g | Healthy Fats: 12g | Carbohydrates: 10g

CHAPTER 6: DESSERTS

Fresh Fruit Salad

Prep Time: 10 minutes | **Cook Time**: 0 minutes | **Per Serving**: 1 serving

Ingredients:

- 1/2 cup strawberries, sliced
- 1/2 cup blueberries
- 1/2 cup pineapple chunks
- 1/2 cup kiwi, peeled and sliced
- 1/2 cup grapes, halved
- 1 tablespoon honey (optional)
- 1 tablespoon fresh mint leaves, chopped (optional)

Instructions:

1. In a large bowl, combine strawberries, blueberries, pineapple chunks, kiwi, and grapes.
2. Drizzle with honey if desired and gently toss to mix.
3. Garnish with fresh mint leaves if desired.
4. Serve immediately and enjoy this colorful and refreshing salad.

Nutritional Value (Approx.): Calories: 150 | Protein: 2g | Fiber: 5g | Healthy Fats: 0g | Carbohydrates: 35g

Berry Parfait with Greek Yogurt

Prep Time: 5 minutes | **Cook Time**: 0 minutes | **Per Serving**: 1 serving

Ingredients:

- 1 cup plain Greek yogurt
- 1/2 cup mixed berries (strawberries, blueberries, raspberries)
- 1 tablespoon honey
- 1/4 cup granola (optional)

Instructions:

1. In a glass or bowl, layer half of the Greek yogurt, followed by half of the mixed berries.
2. Drizzle with half of the honey.
3. Repeat the layers with the remaining yogurt, berries, and honey.
4. Top with granola if desired.
5. Serve immediately and enjoy this delicious and healthy parfait.

Nutritional Value (Approx.): Calories: 250 | Protein: 15g | Fiber: 5g | Healthy Fats: 5g | Carbohydrates: 35g

Chia Seed Pudding with Mango

Prep Time: 10 minutes | **Cook Time**: 0 minutes | Chill Time: 4 hours | **Per Serving**: 1 serving

Ingredients:

- 1/4 cup chia seeds
- 1 cup unsweetened almond milk
- 1 tablespoon maple syrup
- 1/2 teaspoon vanilla extract
- 1/2 cup mango, diced

Instructions:

1. In a bowl, combine chia seeds, almond milk, maple syrup, and vanilla extract. Stir well.
2. Cover and refrigerate for at least 4 hours or overnight, stirring occasionally.
3. Once set, stir the pudding again to break up any clumps.
4. Top with diced mango before serving.
5. Enjoy this creamy and nutritious pudding.

Nutritional Value (Approx.): Calories: 250 | Protein: 6g | Fiber: 12g | Healthy Fats: 10g | Carbohydrates: 35g

Baked Apples with Cinnamon

Prep Time: 10 minutes | **Cook Time**: 25 minutes | **Per Serving**: 1 serving

Ingredients:

- 1 apple, cored and sliced
- 1 tablespoon maple syrup
- 1/2 teaspoon ground cinnamon
- 1 tablespoon chopped walnuts (optional)

Instructions:

1. Preheat the oven to 375°F (190°C).
2. Arrange the apple slices in a baking dish.
3. Drizzle with maple syrup and sprinkle with ground cinnamon.
4. Add chopped walnuts if desired.
5. Bake for 20-25 minutes, until the apples are tender.
6. Serve warm and enjoy this comforting and healthy dessert.

Nutritional Value (Approx.): Calories: 150 | Protein: 1g | Fiber: 4g | Healthy Fats: 2g | Carbohydrates: 35g

Dark Chocolate-Dipped Strawberries

Prep Time: 10 minutes | **Cook Time**: 0 minutes | Chill Time: 15 minutes | **Per Serving**: 1 serving

Ingredients:

- 1/2 cup dark chocolate chips
- 1 teaspoon coconut oil
- 1 cup fresh strawberries

Instructions:

1. In a microwave-safe bowl, combine dark chocolate chips and coconut oil.
2. Microwave in 30-second intervals, stirring each time, until melted and smooth.
3. Dip each strawberry into the melted chocolate, allowing any excess to drip off.
4. Place the dipped strawberries on a parchment-lined baking sheet.
5. Chill in the refrigerator for 15 minutes, or until the chocolate is set.
6. Enjoy this delightful and indulgent treat.

Nutritional Value (Approx.): Calories: 200 | Protein: 2g | Fiber: 4g | Healthy Fats: 12g | Carbohydrates: 25g

Oatmeal Raisin Cookies

Prep Time: 10 minutes | **Cook Time**: 15 minutes | **Per Serving**: 1 serving

Ingredients:

- 1/2 cup rolled oats
- 1/4 cup whole wheat flour
- 1/4 teaspoon baking powder
- 1/4 teaspoon ground cinnamon
- 1/4 cup unsweetened applesauce
- 1/4 cup maple syrup
- 1/4 cup raisins
- 1 teaspoon vanilla extract

Instructions:

1. Preheat the oven to 350°F (175°C).
2. In a bowl, mix together rolled oats, whole wheat flour, baking powder, and ground cinnamon.
3. In another bowl, combine unsweetened applesauce, maple syrup, and vanilla extract.
4. Add the wet ingredients to the dry ingredients and mix until well combined.
5. Stir in the raisins.
6. Drop spoonfuls of the dough onto a parchment-lined baking sheet.
7. Bake for 12-15 minutes, or until the cookies are golden brown.
8. Allow to cool before serving.
9. Enjoy these healthy and chewy cookies.

Nutritional Value (Approx.): Calories: 150 | Protein: 2g | Fiber: 3g | Healthy Fats: 2g | Carbohydrates: 30g

Homemade Applesauce

Prep Time: 10 minutes | **Cook Time**: 25 minutes | **Per Serving**: 1 serving

Ingredients:

- 2 apples, peeled, cored, and chopped
- 1/4 cup water
- 1 tablespoon lemon juice
- 1/2 teaspoon ground cinnamon

Instructions:

1. In a saucepan, combine chopped apples, water, lemon juice, and ground cinnamon.
2. Bring to a boil over medium heat, then reduce heat and simmer for 20-25 minutes, or until the apples are soft.
3. Mash the apples with a fork or blend for a smoother texture.
4. Allow to cool before serving.
5. Enjoy this simple and healthy applesauce.

Nutritional Value (Approx.): Calories: 100 | Protein: 0g | Fiber: 3g | Healthy Fats: 0g | Carbohydrates: 25g

Frozen Banana Bites with Almond Butter

Prep Time: 10 minutes | **Cook Time**: 0 minutes | Freeze Time: 1 hour | **Per Serving**: 1 serving

Ingredients:

- 1 banana, sliced into rounds
- 2 tablespoons almond butter
- 1/4 cup dark chocolate chips
- 1 teaspoon coconut oil

Instructions:

1. Spread almond butter on half of the banana slices.
2. Top with the remaining banana slices to create mini sandwiches.
3. In a microwave-safe bowl, combine dark chocolate chips and coconut oil.
4. Microwave in 30-second intervals, stirring each time, until melted and smooth.
5. Dip each banana sandwich into the melted chocolate, allowing any excess to drip off.
6. Place the dipped banana bites on a parchment-lined baking sheet.
7. Freeze for at least 1 hour, or until the chocolate is set.
8. Enjoy these delicious and nutritious frozen treats.

Nutritional Value (Approx.): Calories: 200 | Protein: 4g | Fiber: 4g | Healthy Fats: 10g | Carbohydrates: 28g

CHAPTER 7: SPECIAL DIETS AND MODIFICATIONS

Low-sodium options

Banana Oat Cookies

Prep Time: 10 minutes | **Cook Time**: 15 minutes | **Per Serving**: 1 serving

Ingredients:

- 1 ripe banana, mashed
- 1 cup rolled oats
- 1/4 cup raisins
- 1/2 teaspoon vanilla extract
- 1/2 teaspoon ground cinnamon

Instructions:

1. Preheat the oven to 350°F (175°C).
2. In a bowl, mix together the mashed banana, rolled oats, raisins, vanilla extract, and ground cinnamon until well combined.
3. Drop spoonfuls of the mixture onto a parchment-lined baking sheet.
4. Bake for 12-15 minutes, or until the cookies are golden brown.
5. Allow to cool before serving.
6. Enjoy these simple and healthy cookies.

Nutritional Value (Approx.): Calories: 120 | Protein: 2g | Fiber: 3g | Healthy Fats: 2g | Carbohydrates: 25g

Raspberry Lemon Sorbet

Prep Time: 10 minutes | **Cook Time**: 0 minutes | Freeze Time: 2 hours | **Per Serving**: 1 serving

Ingredients:

- 2 cups fresh or frozen raspberries
- 1/4 cup lemon juice
- 1/4 cup honey or agave syrup
- 1/2 cup water

Instructions:

1. In a blender, combine raspberries, lemon juice, honey, and water. Blend until smooth.
2. Pour the mixture into a shallow dish and freeze for 2 hours, stirring every 30 minutes to break up ice crystals.
3. Once fully frozen, scoop into bowls and serve.
4. Enjoy this refreshing and tangy sorbet.

Nutritional Value (Approx.): Calories: 100 | Protein: 1g | Fiber: 6g | Healthy Fats: 0g | Carbohydrates: 26g

Poached Pears with Cinnamon

Prep Time: 10 minutes | **Cook Time:** 25 minutes | **Per Serving:** 1 serving

Ingredients:

- 1 pear, peeled, halved, and cored
- 2 cups water
- 1 tablespoon honey
- 1 cinnamon stick

Instructions:

1. In a saucepan, bring water, honey, and the cinnamon stick to a boil.
2. Reduce heat and add the pear halves to the saucepan.
3. Simmer for 20-25 minutes, or until the pears are tender.
4. Remove the pears from the liquid and allow to cool slightly before serving.
5. Enjoy this elegant and fragrant dessert.

Nutritional Value (Approx.): Calories: 120 | Protein: 0g | Fiber: 4g | Healthy Fats: 0g | Carbohydrates: 32g

Pumpkin Spice Muffins

Prep Time: 15 minutes | **Cook Time:** 20 minutes | **Per Serving:** 1 serving

Ingredients:

- 1 cup whole wheat flour
- 1/2 cup rolled oats
- 1/2 cup canned pumpkin puree
- 1/4 cup honey
- 1/4 cup unsweetened applesauce
- 1/2 teaspoon baking soda
- 1/2 teaspoon baking powder
- 1 teaspoon ground cinnamon
- 1/2 teaspoon ground nutmeg
- 1/2 teaspoon ground ginger
- 1/4 teaspoon ground cloves
- 1/4 teaspoon salt

Instructions:

1. Preheat the oven to 350°F (175°C).
2. In a large bowl, mix together the whole wheat flour, rolled oats, baking soda, baking powder, cinnamon, nutmeg, ginger, cloves, and salt.
3. In another bowl, combine the pumpkin puree, honey, and applesauce.
4. Add the wet ingredients to the dry ingredients and mix until just combined.
5. Spoon the batter into a greased or lined muffin tin.

6. Bake for 18-20 minutes, or until a toothpick inserted into the center of a muffin comes out clean.

7. Allow to cool before serving.

8. Enjoy these delicious and healthy muffins.

Nutritional Value (Approx.): Calories: 150 | Protein: 3g | Fiber: 3g | Healthy Fats: 2g | Carbohydrates: 30g

Almond Flour Brownies

Prep Time: 15 minutes | **Cook Time**: 20 minutes | **Per Serving**: 1 serving

Ingredients:

- 1 cup almond flour
- 1/4 cup unsweetened cocoa powder
- 1/2 teaspoon baking soda
- 1/4 teaspoon salt
- 1/4 cup honey or maple syrup
- 1/4 cup coconut oil, melted
- 2 eggs
- 1 teaspoon vanilla extract
- 1/4 cup dark chocolate chips (optional)

Instructions:

1. Preheat the oven to 350°F (175°C).
2. In a large bowl, mix together almond flour, cocoa powder, baking soda, and salt.

3. In another bowl, whisk together honey, melted coconut oil, eggs, and vanilla extract.

4. Add the wet ingredients to the dry ingredients and mix until well combined.

5. Fold in the dark chocolate chips if using.

6. Pour the batter into a greased or lined baking dish.

7. Bake for 18-20 minutes, or until a toothpick inserted into the center comes out clean.

8. Allow to cool before cutting into squares.

9. Enjoy these rich and fudgy brownies.

Nutritional Value (Approx.): Calories: 180 | Protein: 4g | Fiber: 3g | Healthy Fats: 12g | Carbohydrates: 18g

Gluten-free alternatives

Gluten-free alternatives

Baked Pears with Honey and Walnuts

Prep Time: 10 minutes | **Cook Time**: 25 minutes | **Per Serving**: 1 serving

Ingredients:

- 1 pear, halved and cored
- 1 tablespoon honey
- 1 tablespoon chopped walnuts
- 1/2 teaspoon ground cinnamon

Instructions:

1. Preheat the oven to 375°F (190°C).
2. Place the pear halves in a baking dish, cut side up.
3. Drizzle with honey and sprinkle with chopped walnuts and ground cinnamon.
4. Bake for 25 minutes, or until the pears are tender.
5. Allow to cool slightly before serving.
6. Enjoy this warm and nutritious dessert.

Nutritional Value (Approx.): Calories: 150 | Protein: 1g | Fiber: 4g | Healthy Fats: 5g | Carbohydrates: 30g

Chia Seed Pudding with Vanilla and Berries

Prep Time: 10 minutes | **Cook Time**: 0 minutes | Chill Time: 4 hours | **Per Serving**: 1 serving

Ingredients:

- 1/4 cup chia seeds
- 1 cup unsweetened almond milk
- 1 tablespoon maple syrup
- 1/2 teaspoon vanilla extract
- 1/2 cup mixed berries (strawberries, blueberries, raspberries)

Instructions:

1. In a bowl, combine chia seeds, almond milk, maple syrup, and vanilla extract. Stir well.
2. Cover and refrigerate for at least 4 hours or overnight, stirring occasionally.
3. Once set, stir the pudding again to break up any clumps.
4. Top with mixed berries before serving.
5. Enjoy this creamy and nutritious pudding.

Nutritional Value (Approx.): Calories: 250 | Protein: 6g | Fiber: 12g | Healthy Fats: 10g | Carbohydrates: 35g

Chocolate Avocado Mousse

Prep Time: 10 minutes | **Cook Time**: 0 minutes | Chill Time: 30 minutes | **Per Serving**: 1 serving

Ingredients:

- 1 ripe avocado, peeled and pitted
- 2 tablespoons unsweetened cocoa powder
- 2 tablespoons honey or maple syrup
- 1/4 teaspoon vanilla extract
- Pinch of sea salt

Instructions:

1. In a blender or food processor, combine avocado, cocoa powder, honey, vanilla extract, and sea salt.
2. Blend until smooth and creamy.
3. Spoon the mousse into a bowl and chill in the refrigerator for at least 30 minutes before serving.
4. Enjoy this rich and healthy dessert.

Nutritional Value (Approx.): Calories: 200 | Protein: 2g | Fiber: 7g | Healthy Fats: 14g | Carbohydrates: 20g

Gluten-Free Lemon Bars

Prep Time: 20 minutes | **Cook Time**: 25 minutes | **Per Serving**: 1 serving

Ingredients:

- 1 cup almond flour
- 1/4 cup coconut oil, melted
- 1/4 cup honey or maple syrup
- 2 eggs
- 1/4 cup lemon juice
- 1 tablespoon lemon zest
- 1/4 cup honey or maple syrup (for filling)
- 2 tablespoons coconut flour

Instructions:

1. Preheat the oven to 350°F (175°C).
2. In a bowl, mix almond flour, melted coconut oil, and 1/4 cup honey until combined.
3. Press the mixture into a greased or lined baking dish to form the crust.
4. Bake for 10 minutes, then remove from the oven.
5. In another bowl, whisk together eggs, lemon juice, lemon zest, 1/4 cup honey, and coconut flour.
6. Pour the lemon mixture over the baked crust.
7. Bake for an additional 15 minutes, or until the filling is set.
8. Allow to cool before cutting into bars.
9. Enjoy these tangy and refreshing lemon bars.

Nutritional Value (Approx.): Calories: 180 | Protein: 4g | Fiber: 3g | Healthy Fats: 12g | Carbohydrates: 16g

Mango Sticky Rice

Prep Time: 10 minutes | **Cook Time:** 30 minutes | **Per Serving:** 1 serving

Ingredients:

- 1/2 cup glutinous rice
- 1/2 cup coconut milk
- 2 tablespoons sugar
- 1/4 teaspoon salt
- 1 ripe mango, peeled and sliced

Instructions:

1. Rinse the glutinous rice under cold water until the water runs clear.
2. In a pot, combine the rinsed rice with 1 cup of water. Bring to a boil, then reduce heat to low, cover, and simmer for 20 minutes, or until the water is absorbed and the rice is tender.
3. In a separate saucepan, heat the coconut milk, sugar, and salt over low heat, stirring until the sugar dissolves.
4. Remove the coconut milk mixture from heat and stir in the cooked rice. Cover and let sit for 10 minutes to absorb the flavors.
5. Serve the sticky rice with sliced mango on top.
6. Enjoy this sweet and tropical dessert.

Nutritional Value (Approx.): Calories: 250 | Protein: 3g | Fiber: 2g | Healthy Fats: 10g | Carbohydrates: 40g

Vegetarian and vegan modifications

Raw Vegan Cheesecake

Prep Time: 20 minutes | **Cook Time**: 0 minutes | Chill Time: 4 hours | **Per Serving**: 1 serving

Ingredients:

- 1 cup raw cashews (soaked overnight)
- 1/4 cup coconut oil, melted
- 1/4 cup maple syrup
- 1/4 cup lemon juice
- 1 teaspoon vanilla extract
- 1 cup mixed berries (for topping)

Instructions:

1. Drain and rinse the soaked cashews.
2. In a blender, combine cashews, coconut oil, maple syrup, lemon juice, and vanilla extract. Blend until smooth.
3. Pour the mixture into a springform pan and spread evenly.
4. Chill in the refrigerator for at least 4 hours or until set.
5. Top with mixed berries before serving.
6. Enjoy this creamy and delicious raw vegan cheesecake.

Nutritional Value (Approx.): Calories: 250 | Protein: 6g | Fiber: 2g | Healthy Fats: 18g | Carbohydrates: 20g

Vegan Pumpkin Pie

Prep Time: 15 minutes | **Cook Time**: 45 minutes | **Per Serving**: 1 serving

Ingredients:

- 1 cup canned pumpkin puree
- 1/2 cup coconut milk
- 1/4 cup maple syrup
- 2 tablespoons cornstarch
- 1 teaspoon ground cinnamon
- 1/2 teaspoon ground ginger
- 1/4 teaspoon ground cloves
- 1/4 teaspoon salt
- 1 vegan pie crust

Instructions:

1. Preheat the oven to 350°F (175°C).
2. In a bowl, combine pumpkin puree, coconut milk, maple syrup, cornstarch, cinnamon, ginger, cloves, and salt. Mix until smooth.
3. Pour the mixture into the vegan pie crust.
4. Bake for 45 minutes, or until the filling is set.
5. Allow to cool before slicing.
6. Enjoy this flavorful and comforting vegan pumpkin pie.

Nutritional Value (Approx.): Calories: 220 | Protein: 3g | Fiber: 3g | Healthy Fats: 12g | Carbohydrates: 25g

Vegan Chocolate Truffles

Prep Time: 15 minutes | **Cook Time**: 0 minutes | Chill Time: 1 hour | **Per Serving**: 1 serving

Ingredients:

- 1 cup dates, pitted
- 1/2 cup raw almonds
- 1/4 cup unsweetened cocoa powder
- 1 teaspoon vanilla extract
- Pinch of sea salt
- Unsweetened shredded coconut (for rolling)

Instructions:

1. In a food processor, combine dates, almonds, cocoa powder, vanilla extract, and sea salt. Process until the mixture forms a sticky dough.
2. Roll the dough into small balls.
3. Roll each ball in shredded coconut to coat.
4. Chill in the refrigerator for at least 1 hour before serving.
5. Enjoy these rich and indulgent vegan chocolate truffles.

Nutritional Value (Approx.): Calories: 100 | Protein: 2g | Fiber: 3g | Healthy Fats: 5g | Carbohydrates: 15g

Vegan Lemon Poppy Seed Muffins

Prep Time: 15 minutes | **Cook Time:** 20 minutes | **Per Serving:** 1 serving

Ingredients:

- 1 1/2 cups whole wheat flour
- 1/2 cup coconut sugar
- 1/4 cup poppy seeds
- 1 teaspoon baking soda
- 1/2 teaspoon baking powder
- 1/4 teaspoon salt
- 1 cup almond milk
- 1/4 cup coconut oil, melted
- 1/4 cup lemon juice
- 1 tablespoon lemon zest
- 1 teaspoon vanilla extract

Instructions:

1. Preheat the oven to 350°F (175°C).
2. In a large bowl, combine whole wheat flour, coconut sugar, poppy seeds, baking soda, baking powder, and salt.
3. In another bowl, mix almond milk, melted coconut oil, lemon juice, lemon zest, and vanilla extract.
4. Add the wet ingredients to the dry ingredients and mix until just combined.
5. Spoon the batter into a greased or lined muffin tin.

6. Bake for 18-20 minutes, or until a toothpick inserted into the center of a muffin comes out clean.

7. Allow to cool before serving.

8. Enjoy these light and zesty vegan muffins.

Nutritional Value (Approx.): Calories: 180 | Protein: 3g | Fiber: 2g | Healthy Fats: 8g | Carbohydrates: 25g

Vegan Peanut Butter Cups

Prep Time: 15 minutes | **Cook Time**: 0 minutes | Chill Time: 30 minutes | **Per Serving**: 1 serving

Ingredients:

- 1/2 cup natural peanut butter
- 1/4 cup coconut oil, melted
- 1/4 cup maple syrup
- 1 cup vegan dark chocolate chips
- Sea salt (optional)

Instructions:

1. In a bowl, mix together peanut butter, melted coconut oil, and maple syrup until smooth.

2. In a separate bowl, melt the dark chocolate chips in the microwave or over a double boiler.

3. Spoon a layer of melted chocolate into the bottom of mini muffin liners.

4. Add a spoonful of the peanut butter mixture on top of the chocolate layer.

5. Cover with another layer of melted chocolate.

6. Sprinkle with sea salt if desired.
7. Chill in the refrigerator for at least 30 minutes before serving.
8. Enjoy these creamy and delicious vegan peanut butter cups.

Nutritional Value (Approx.): Calories: 180 | Protein: 4g | Fiber: 2g | Healthy Fats: 14g | Carbohydrates: 14g

Dairy-free substitutions

Vegan Chocolate Pudding

Prep Time: 10 minutes | **Cook Time**: 0 minutes | Chill Time: 2 hours | **Per Serving**: 1 serving

Ingredients:

- 1 ripe avocado, peeled and pitted
- 1/4 cup unsweetened cocoa powder
- 1/4 cup maple syrup
- 1/4 cup almond milk
- 1 teaspoon vanilla extract
- Pinch of sea salt

Instructions:

1. In a blender, combine avocado, cocoa powder, maple syrup, almond milk, vanilla extract, and sea salt.
2. Blend until smooth and creamy.
3. Spoon the pudding into serving bowls.
4. Chill in the refrigerator for at least 2 hours before serving.

5. Enjoy this rich and creamy vegan chocolate pudding.

Nutritional Value (Approx.): Calories: 220 | Protein: 3g | Fiber: 6g | Healthy Fats: 14g | Carbohydrates: 25g

Coconut Milk Ice Cream

Prep Time: 15 minutes | **Cook Time:** 0 minutes | Freeze Time: 4 hours | **Per Serving:** 1 serving

Ingredients:

- 2 cups full-fat coconut milk
- 1/2 cup maple syrup
- 1 teaspoon vanilla extract
- Pinch of sea salt

Instructions:

1. In a bowl, whisk together coconut milk, maple syrup, vanilla extract, and sea salt until well combined.
2. Pour the mixture into an ice cream maker and churn according to the manufacturer's instructions.
3. Transfer the ice cream to a container and freeze for at least 4 hours, or until firm.
4. Scoop and serve.
5. Enjoy this creamy and dairy-free coconut milk ice cream.

Nutritional Value (Approx.): Calories: 250 | Protein: 2g | Fiber: 1g | Healthy Fats: 20g | Carbohydrates: 20g

Date and Nut Energy Balls

Prep Time: 15 minutes | **Cook Time:** 0 minutes | Chill Time: 30 minutes | **Per Serving:** 1 serving

Ingredients:

- 1 cup dates, pitted
- 1/2 cup almonds
- 1/2 cup walnuts
- 1 tablespoon chia seeds
- 1 tablespoon flaxseeds
- 1 teaspoon vanilla extract
- Pinch of sea salt

Instructions:

1. In a food processor, combine dates, almonds, walnuts, chia seeds, flaxseeds, vanilla extract, and sea salt. Process until the mixture forms a sticky dough.
2. Roll the dough into small balls.
3. Place the energy balls on a baking sheet and chill in the refrigerator for at least 30 minutes before serving.
4. Enjoy these nutritious and energy-boosting snacks.

Nutritional Value (Approx.): Calories: 150 | Protein: 3g | Fiber: 4g | Healthy Fats: 10g | Carbohydrates: 15g

Dairy-Free Apple Crisp

Prep Time: 15 minutes | **Cook Time**: 30 minutes | **Per Serving**: 1 serving

Ingredients:

- 3 cups apples, peeled and sliced
- 1/2 cup rolled oats
- 1/4 cup almond flour
- 1/4 cup coconut sugar
- 1/4 cup coconut oil, melted
- 1 teaspoon ground cinnamon
- 1/4 teaspoon ground nutmeg
- 1/4 teaspoon salt

Instructions:

1. Preheat the oven to 350°F (175°C).
2. In a bowl, toss the sliced apples with 1/4 teaspoon of cinnamon and set aside.
3. In another bowl, mix together rolled oats, almond flour, coconut sugar, melted coconut oil, the remaining cinnamon, nutmeg, and salt.
4. Place the apples in a baking dish and spread the oat mixture on top.
5. Bake for 30 minutes, or until the topping is golden brown and the apples are tender.
6. Allow to cool slightly before serving.
7. Enjoy this warm and comforting dairy-free apple crisp.

Nutritional Value (Approx.): Calories: 200 | Protein: 2g | Fiber: 4g | Healthy Fats: 10g | Carbohydrates: 25g

Avocado Lime Sorbet

Prep Time: 15 minutes | **Cook Time**: 0 minutes | Chill Time: 4 hours | **Per Serving**: 1 serving

Ingredients:

- 2 ripe avocados, peeled and pitted
- 1/2 cup lime juice
- 1/4 cup coconut milk
- 1/4 cup maple syrup
- 1 teaspoon lime zest

Instructions:

1. In a blender, combine avocados, lime juice, coconut milk, maple syrup, and lime zest. Blend until smooth.
2. Pour the mixture into a container and freeze for at least 4 hours, or until firm.
3. Scoop and serve.
4. Enjoy this refreshing and creamy avocado lime sorbet.

Nutritional Value (Approx.): Calories: 180 | Protein: 2g | Fiber: 6g | Healthy Fats: 14g | Carbohydrates: 18g

CHAPTER 8: FITNESS AND LIFESTYLE TIPS

Regular physical activity is a crucial component of managing congestive heart failure (CHF) and promoting overall heart health. Incorporating exercise into your routine can help improve cardiovascular function, manage weight, and enhance overall well-being. Here's how to effectively integrate exercise into your lifestyle:

1. Understanding the Role of Exercise

Exercise plays a vital role in managing CHF by improving heart function, increasing stamina, and reducing symptoms. It can help:

- **Improve Cardiovascular Health:** Strengthens the heart muscle and improves circulation.
- **Manage Weight:** Aids in maintaining a healthy weight, which can reduce the strain on the heart.
- **Enhance Energy Levels:** Boosts overall energy and reduces feelings of fatigue.
- **Reduce Stress:** Helps lower stress levels and improve mental well-being.

2. Types of Exercise

2.1. Aerobic Exercise

- **Why:** Improves cardiovascular fitness and endurance.
- **Examples:** Walking, cycling, swimming, or using an elliptical machine.
- **Tips:** Aim for moderate-intensity aerobic exercise for at least 150 minutes per week, or 30 minutes most days of the week. Start slowly and gradually increase duration and intensity.

2.2. Strength Training

- **Why:** Builds muscle strength, improves metabolism, and supports joint health.

- **Examples:** Light weight lifting, resistance bands, body-weight exercises like squats or lunges.

- **Tips:** Incorporate strength training exercises 2-3 times per week. Focus on major muscle groups and use light weights to start, gradually increasing as strength improves.

2.3. Flexibility and Stretching

- **Why:** Enhances range of motion and reduces muscle tension.

- **Examples:** Stretching exercises, yoga, or Pilates.

- **Tips:** Perform stretching exercises daily or at least 3 times per week. Include stretches for major muscle groups and hold each stretch for 15-30 seconds.

2.4. Balance and Coordination

- **Why:** Improves stability and reduces the risk of falls.

- **Examples:** Balance exercises, tai chi, or simple coordination drills.

- **Tips:** Incorporate balance and coordination exercises 2-3 times per week, especially if you have concerns about balance or fall risk.

3. Starting an Exercise Routine

3.1. Consult with Your Healthcare Provider

- **Why:** Ensures that your exercise plan is safe and appropriate for your condition.

- **Tips:** Discuss your exercise goals and any limitations with your healthcare provider. Obtain clearance and specific recommendations based on your health status.

3.2. Set Realistic Goals

- **Why:** Helps maintain motivation and track progress.

- **Tips:** Set achievable short-term and long-term goals. Start with smaller goals, such as walking for 10 minutes a day, and gradually increase the duration and intensity.

3.3. Create a Routine

- **Why:** Establishes consistency and makes exercise a regular part of your day.
- **Tips:** Choose times for exercise that fit your schedule. Consider incorporating physical activity into daily routines, such as walking after meals or using stairs instead of elevators.

3.4. Choose Enjoyable Activities

- **Why:** Increases adherence and makes exercise more enjoyable.
- **Tips:** Select activities you enjoy, whether it's dancing, gardening, or playing a sport. Engaging in activities you like can make it easier to stick to your routine.

3.5. Monitor Your Progress

- **Why:** Helps track improvements and stay motivated.
- **Tips:** Keep a log of your exercise sessions, noting the type, duration, and intensity of each workout. Use fitness apps or journals to track progress and celebrate achievements.

4. Safety and Considerations

4.1. Listen to Your Body

- **Why:** Prevents overexertion and injury.
- **Tips:** Pay attention to how your body responds to exercise. Stop and seek medical advice if you experience unusual symptoms such as chest pain, shortness of breath, or dizziness.

4.2. Stay Hydrated

- **Why:** Maintains proper hydration and supports overall health.

- **Tips:** Drink water before, during, and after exercise. Avoid excessive caffeine or sugary drinks.

4.3. Wear Appropriate Clothing and Gear

- **Why:** Ensures comfort and safety during exercise.
- **Tips:** Wear supportive, well-fitting footwear and comfortable clothing suitable for the activity. Consider using heart rate monitors or pedometers to track your activity.

4.4. Adapt Exercises as Needed

- **Why:** Accommodates any physical limitations or health changes.
- **Tips:** Modify exercises to suit your current fitness level and any physical limitations. Use supportive equipment or adjust intensity as needed.

4.5. Include Rest and Recovery

- **Why:** Allows the body to recover and prevents overtraining.
- **Tips:** Incorporate rest days into your routine to allow muscles to recover. Ensure you get adequate sleep and rest between exercise sessions.

Benefits of Physical Activity for CHF Patients

Engaging in regular physical activity provides numerous advantages for individuals managing congestive heart failure (CHF). Here are some key benefits:

Improved Cardiovascular Function

- Regular exercise strengthens the heart muscle, allowing it to pump blood more effectively. This enhances cardiac output and improves the heart's ability to handle physical stress.

- Exercise promotes better blood flow throughout the body, which helps reduce symptoms such as swelling and fluid retention by improving venous return.

Better Management of Symptoms

- Physical activity improves lung function and the efficiency of the respiratory system, helping patients breathe more easily and manage shortness of breath during daily activities.

- Regular exercise boosts overall stamina and energy levels, reducing feelings of fatigue and improving the ability to perform daily tasks.

Weight Management

- Exercise helps burn calories and manage body weight, assisting in maintaining a healthy weight. This reduces the strain on the heart and can improve overall heart function.

- Physical activity enhances metabolic processes, helping manage comorbid conditions such as diabetes and hypertension, which can affect heart health.

Enhanced Physical Fitness

- Regular exercise builds muscle strength and cardiovascular endurance, improving overall physical fitness and making it easier to engage in daily activities. It also reduces feelings of weakness.

- Exercise routines often include stretching and balance exercises, which enhance flexibility and balance, helping to prevent falls and improve mobility.

Improved Psychological Well-being

- Exercise stimulates the release of endorphins and other mood-enhancing chemicals, helping alleviate stress, anxiety, and symptoms of depression, contributing to better mental health.

- Physical activity can boost self-esteem and overall mood, providing a sense of accomplishment and contributing to a more positive outlook on life.

Better Sleep Quality

- Regular exercise helps regulate sleep cycles, promoting deeper and more restful sleep, which is important for overall health and recovery.

- Exercise helps expend energy and reduce anxiety, which can lead to fewer episodes of insomnia and better sleep quality.

Enhanced Overall Health

- Physical activity supports various aspects of health, reducing the risk of complications related to CHF, such as hospitalizations and exacerbations.

- Regular exercise contributes to a healthier lifestyle, which may improve life expectancy by enhancing overall health and reducing the risk of cardiovascular events.

Personalized Benefits

- Exercise programs can be tailored to individual needs and abilities, providing a safe and effective way to manage CHF symptoms based on personal health conditions and fitness levels.

- Professional guidance ensures exercises are safe and beneficial, helping in designing a suitable exercise plan and monitoring progress for better health outcomes.

Gentle Exercises and Routines for CHF Patients

For individuals managing congestive heart failure (CHF), gentle exercises and routines can be highly effective in improving overall health while minimizing strain on the heart. Here are some suitable exercises and routines:

1. Walking

- **Description:** Walking is a low-impact, moderate-intensity exercise that can be easily adjusted to match fitness levels.
- **Routine:** Start with short walks of 10-15 minutes, gradually increasing the duration as tolerated. Aim for 3-5 times per week. Walking indoors or on a treadmill can be beneficial if outdoor conditions are not favorable.

2. Chair Exercises

- **Description:** Chair exercises are ideal for those with limited mobility or who need additional support.
- **Routine:** While seated, perform leg lifts, seated marches, and arm circles. These exercises help improve circulation, muscle strength, and flexibility. Aim for 10-15 minutes, 2-3 times per day.

3. Stretching

- **Description:** Stretching helps maintain flexibility and prevent muscle stiffness.
- **Routine:** Perform gentle stretches for major muscle groups, such as hamstrings, calves, and shoulders. Hold each stretch for 15-30 seconds and repeat 2-3 times. Incorporate stretching into your daily routine or as part of a warm-up before other exercises.

4. Seated Strength Training

- **Description:** Using light weights or resistance bands while seated can enhance muscle strength without excessive strain.

- **Routine:** Perform exercises such as bicep curls, seated rows, and leg extensions. Use light weights or resistance bands and aim for 1-2 sets of 10-15 repetitions for each exercise, 2-3 times per week.

5. Water Aerobics

- **Description:** Water aerobics provides a full-body workout with minimal impact on the joints.
- **Routine:** Join a water aerobics class or perform exercises in the pool, such as leg lifts, water walking, and arm movements. Aim for 20-30 minutes, 2-3 times per week. The buoyancy of the water reduces the risk of injury and supports easier movement.

6. Tai Chi

- **Description:** Tai Chi is a gentle, flowing exercise that improves balance, flexibility, and mental relaxation.
- **Routine:** Practice Tai Chi sessions or follow a video guide to perform slow, deliberate movements. Aim for 20-30 minutes, 2-3 times per week. Tai Chi can be practiced indoors or in a calm outdoor setting.

7. Breathing Exercises

- **Description:** Breathing exercises help improve lung function and reduce stress.
- **Routine:** Practice deep breathing techniques, such as diaphragmatic breathing or pursed-lip breathing. Spend 5-10 minutes each day focusing on slow, deep breaths. Breathing exercises can be done seated or lying down.

8. Range-of-Motion Exercises

- **Description:** These exercises help maintain joint flexibility and reduce stiffness.
- **Routine:** Perform gentle range-of-motion exercises, such as shoulder circles, ankle rolls, and wrist flexions. Aim for 10-15 minutes, 2-3 times per day, particularly if you have limited mobility.

9. Functional Activities

- **Description:** Engaging in functional activities, such as gardening or light housework, can provide beneficial movement and exercise.

- **Routine:** Incorporate light activities into your daily routine, focusing on tasks that involve movement and light exertion. Be mindful of pacing yourself and taking breaks as needed.

10. Mindful Movement

- **Description:** Mindful movement practices, such as gentle yoga or stretching, can improve flexibility and relaxation.

- **Routine:** Follow a gentle yoga routine or stretching sequence designed for heart health. Aim for 15-20 minutes, 2-3 times per week. Focus on slow, controlled movements and deep breathing.

When incorporating gentle exercises into your routine, consider the following tips:

- **Consult with Your Healthcare Provider:** Before starting any new exercise program, discuss it with your healthcare provider to ensure it is safe and appropriate for your condition.

- **Listen to Your Body:** Pay attention to how your body responds to exercise. Stop and seek medical advice if you experience unusual symptoms such as chest pain, dizziness, or shortness of breath.

- **Start Slowly:** Begin with lower intensity and gradually increase the duration and intensity of your exercise as tolerated.

- **Stay Hydrated:** Drink water before, during, and after exercise to stay hydrated.

- **Warm Up and Cool Down:** Include a warm-up and cool-down period in your exercise routine to prevent injury and promote recovery.

Tips for Staying Active Safely with CHF

Engaging in physical activity is beneficial for managing congestive heart failure (CHF), but it's crucial to approach exercise with care to ensure safety and effectiveness. Here are some tips for staying active safely:

1. Consult with Your Healthcare Provider

- **Why:** Ensures that your exercise plan is safe and tailored to your individual health needs.

- **Tips:** Discuss your exercise goals, any limitations, and get medical clearance before starting a new exercise regimen. Your provider can offer specific recommendations based on your health status.

2. Start Slowly and Progress Gradually

- **Why:** Allows your body to adapt to increased physical activity without excessive strain.

- **Tips:** Begin with low-intensity exercises and gradually increase the duration and intensity. Start with 5-10 minutes of activity and build up as tolerated.

3. Choose Low-Impact Activities

- **Why:** Reduces stress on joints and minimizes the risk of injury.

- **Tips:** Opt for low-impact exercises such as walking, swimming, or using an elliptical machine. Avoid high-impact activities that could place excessive stress on the heart and joints.

4. Monitor Your Symptoms

- **Why:** Helps identify any adverse effects or signs of overexertion.

- **Tips:** Pay attention to how your body responds to exercise. Stop and seek medical advice if you experience symptoms such as chest pain, severe shortness of breath, dizziness, or unusual fatigue.

5. Stay Hydrated

- **Why:** Prevents dehydration and supports overall health.

- **Tips:** Drink water before, during, and after exercise. Avoid excessive consumption of caffeinated or sugary beverages.

6. Incorporate Warm-Up and Cool-Down

- **Why:** Helps prepare your body for exercise and promotes recovery.

- **Tips:** Spend 5-10 minutes warming up with gentle movements or stretching before starting your workout. Similarly, cool down with stretching and deep breathing to help relax your muscles and lower your heart rate.

7. Use Proper Equipment

- **Why:** Ensures comfort and safety during exercise.

- **Tips:** Wear supportive, well-fitting footwear and comfortable clothing suitable for your chosen activity. Use any recommended aids or equipment, such as heart rate monitors, if advised by your healthcare provider.

8. Listen to Your Body

- **Why:** Prevents overexertion and minimizes the risk of injury.

- **Tips:** Exercise at a pace that feels comfortable and manageable. If you feel overly fatigued or experience any discomfort, take a break and reassess your activity level.

9. Follow a Structured Exercise Program

- **Why:** Provides a balanced approach to physical activity and ensures safety.

- **Tips:** Consider working with a physical therapist or exercise specialist who can design a structured exercise program tailored to your needs and monitor your

- progress.

10. Incorporate Rest Days

- **Why:** Allows your body to recover and reduces the risk of overtraining.
- **Tips:** Include rest days in your exercise routine to prevent excessive strain on your body. Alternate between days of activity and rest or low-intensity exercises.

11. Set Realistic Goals

- **Why:** Helps maintain motivation and avoid overexertion.
- **Tips:** Set achievable and specific goals for your exercise routine. Focus on gradual progress and celebrate small milestones to stay motivated.

12. Stay Consistent

- **Why:** Consistent physical activity supports long-term health benefits.
- **Tips:** Aim to incorporate exercise into your daily or weekly routine. Consistency is key to achieving and maintaining improvements in heart health and overall well-being.

13. Adapt Exercises as Needed

- **Why:** Ensures that exercises are appropriate for your current fitness level and health condition.
- **Tips:** Modify exercises to accommodate any physical limitations or changes in your health. Use supportive equipment or adjust intensity as necessary.

14. Focus on Enjoyable Activities

- **Why:** Increases adherence and makes exercise more enjoyable.
- **Tips:** Choose activities you enjoy and find fulfilling. Engaging in enjoyable exercises can make it easier to maintain a regular activity routine.

Techniques for Relaxation and Mindfulness

Practicing relaxation and mindfulness techniques can be highly beneficial for individuals with congestive heart failure (CHF) by reducing stress, improving mental health, and enhancing overall well-being. Here are some effective techniques:

1. Deep Breathing Exercises

- **Why:** Promotes relaxation and reduces stress by slowing the heart rate and lowering blood pressure.

- **How:** Sit or lie down in a comfortable position. Inhale deeply through your nose, allowing your abdomen to rise. Exhale slowly through your mouth. Repeat for 5-10 minutes, focusing on the rhythm of your breath.

2. Progressive Muscle Relaxation

- **Why:** Helps release tension and promotes physical relaxation by progressively tensing and relaxing different muscle groups.

- **How:** Start with your toes and work your way up to your head. Tense each muscle group for 5-10 seconds, then slowly release the tension. Notice the difference between tension and relaxation.

3. Mindfulness Meditation

- **Why:** Enhances mental clarity, reduces stress, and improves emotional well-being by focusing on the present moment.

- **How:** Sit comfortably and close your eyes. Focus on your breath, noticing each inhale and exhale. When your mind wanders, gently bring your focus back to your breath. Practice for 5-20 minutes daily.

4. Guided Imagery

- **Why:** Reduces stress and promotes relaxation by visualizing peaceful and calming scenes.

- **How:** Close your eyes and imagine a serene place, such as a beach or forest. Use all your senses to make the image as vivid as possible. Spend 5-10 minutes immersed in this scene, allowing yourself to feel calm and relaxed.

5. Body Scan Meditation

- **Why:** Increases awareness of bodily sensations and promotes relaxation by systematically focusing on different parts of the body.
- **How:** Lie down or sit comfortably. Close your eyes and bring your attention to your toes, slowly moving up to your head. Notice any sensations, tension, or areas of relaxation without judgment. Spend 10-20 minutes scanning your entire body.

6. Yoga

- **Why:** Combines physical postures, breathing exercises, and meditation to improve flexibility, reduce stress, and promote overall well-being.
- **How:** Follow a gentle yoga routine or attend a class designed for beginners or those with health conditions. Focus on slow, controlled movements and deep breathing. Practice for 20-30 minutes, 2-3 times per week.

7. Tai Chi

- **Why:** Enhances balance, reduces stress, and promotes relaxation through slow, flowing movements and deep breathing.
- **How:** Join a Tai Chi class or follow a video guide to learn the basic movements. Practice for 20-30 minutes, 2-3 times per week, focusing on the smooth and deliberate transitions between poses.

8. Aromatherapy

- **Why:** Uses essential oils to promote relaxation and reduce stress through the sense of smell.

- **How:** Use a diffuser to disperse calming essential oils, such as lavender, chamomile, or bergamot, into the air. Alternatively, apply a few drops to a cotton ball and inhale deeply, or add essential oils to a warm bath.

9. Journaling

- **Why:** Provides an outlet for expressing thoughts and emotions, reducing stress and promoting mental clarity.
- **How:** Set aside time each day to write about your thoughts, feelings, and experiences. Focus on expressing yourself freely without judgment. Use prompts if needed, such as "What am I grateful for today?" or "What challenges did I face today?"

10. Listening to Music

- **Why:** Reduces stress and promotes relaxation by engaging the auditory senses.
- **How:** Choose calming music, such as classical, nature sounds, or instrumental tracks. Listen for 10-20 minutes, focusing on the music and allowing yourself to relax.

11. Spending Time in Nature

- **Why:** Promotes relaxation and reduces stress by connecting with the natural environment.
- **How:** Spend time outdoors in a park, garden, or nature reserve. Engage in gentle activities such as walking or simply sitting and observing the surroundings. Focus on the sights, sounds, and smells of nature.

12. Practicing Gratitude

- **Why:** Enhances mental well-being and reduces stress by focusing on positive aspects of life.
- **How:** Each day, write down three things you are grateful for. Reflect on these positive aspects and how they contribute to your well-being.

CHAPTER 9: 28-Day Meal Plan for Congestive Heart Failure

Week 1

Day 1

- Breakfast: Smoothie with Spinach and Berries
- Lunch: Grilled Chicken Salad with Mixed Greens
- Snack: Hummus with Veggie Sticks
- Dinner: Baked Cod with Asparagus and Lemon
- Dessert: Fresh Fruit Salad

Day 2

- Breakfast: Chia Seed Pudding
- Lunch: Lentil and Vegetable Soup
- Snack: Apple Slices with Almond Butter
- Dinner: Turkey and Vegetable Stir-Fry
- Dessert: Berry Parfait with Greek Yogurt

Day 3

- Breakfast: Avocado Toast
- Lunch: Quinoa and Black Bean Salad
- Snack: Greek Yogurt with Honey and Walnuts
- Dinner: Stuffed Bell Peppers with Quinoa and Black Beans
- Dessert: Chia Seed Pudding with Mango

Day 4

- Breakfast: Greek Yogurt Parfait
- Lunch: Turkey and Avocado Wrap
- Snack: Spiced Chickpea Crunch
- Dinner: Roasted Chicken with Sweet Potatoes and Brussels Sprouts
- Dessert: Baked Apples with Cinnamon

Day 5

- Breakfast: Oatmeal with Berries and Almonds
- Lunch: Grilled Chicken Salad with Mixed Greens
- Snack: Baked Sweet Potato Chips
- Dinner: Spinach and Ricotta Stuffed Shells
- Dessert: Dark Chocolate-Dipped Strawberries

Day 6

- Breakfast: Quinoa Breakfast Bowl
- Lunch: Lentil and Vegetable Soup
- Snack: Caprese Skewers (Cherry Tomatoes, Basil, and Mozzarella)
- Dinner: Slow Cooker Chicken Stew
- Dessert: Oatmeal Raisin Cookies

Day 7

- Breakfast: Blueberry Buckwheat Pancakes
- Lunch: Quinoa and Black Bean Salad
- Snack: Avocado and Black Bean Salsa

- Dinner: Lentil and Vegetable Shepherd's Pie
- Dessert: Homemade Applesauce

Week 2

Day 8

- Breakfast: Spinach and Mushroom Egg White Omelette
- Lunch: Turkey and Avocado Wrap
- Snack: Cucumber and Tomato Salad
- Dinner: Herb-Crusted Pork Tenderloin with Steamed Broccoli
- Dessert: Frozen Banana Bites with Almond Butter

Day 9

- Breakfast: Smoothie with Spinach and Berries
- Lunch: Baked Cod with Asparagus and Lemon
- Snack: Hummus with Veggie Sticks
- Dinner: Stuffed Bell Peppers with Brown Rice and Vegetables
- Dessert: Banana Oat Cookies

Day 10

- Breakfast: Chia Seed Pudding
- Lunch: Grilled Salmon with Asparagus
- Snack: Apple Slices with Almond Butter
- Dinner: Chicken and Quinoa Stir-Fry
- Dessert: Raspberry Lemon Sorbet

Day 11

- Breakfast: Avocado Toast
- Lunch: Mediterranean Chickpea Salad
- Snack: Greek Yogurt with Honey and Walnuts
- Dinner: Spinach and Ricotta Stuffed Shells
- Dessert: Poached Pears with Cinnamon

Day 12

- Breakfast: Greek Yogurt Parfait
- Lunch: Grilled Chicken Salad with Mixed Greens
- Snack: Spiced Chickpea Crunch
- Dinner: Slow Cooker Chicken Stew
- Dessert: Pumpkin Spice Muffins

Day 13

- Breakfast: Oatmeal with Berries and Almonds
- Lunch: Lentil and Vegetable Soup
- Snack: Baked Sweet Potato Chips
- Dinner: Lentil and Vegetable Shepherd's Pie
- Dessert: Almond Flour Brownies

Day 14

- Breakfast: Quinoa Breakfast Bowl
- Lunch: Quinoa and Black Bean Salad
- Snack: Caprese Skewers (Cherry Tomatoes, Basil, and Mozzarella)
- Dinner: Herb-Crusted Pork Tenderloin with Steamed Broccoli

- Dessert: Baked Pears with Honey and Walnuts

Week 3

Day 15

- Breakfast: Blueberry Buckwheat Pancakes
- Lunch: Turkey and Avocado Wrap
- Snack: Avocado and Black Bean Salsa
- Dinner: Baked Cod with Asparagus and Lemon
- Dessert: Chia Seed Pudding with Vanilla and Berries

Day 16

- Breakfast: Spinach and Mushroom Egg White Omelette
- Lunch: Grilled Chicken Salad with Mixed Greens
- Snack: Cucumber and Tomato Salad
- Dinner: Turkey and Vegetable Stir-Fry
- Dessert: Chocolate Avocado Mousse

Day 17

- Breakfast: Smoothie with Spinach and Berries
- Lunch: Lentil and Vegetable Soup
- Snack: Hummus with Veggie Sticks
- Dinner: Stuffed Bell Peppers with Quinoa and Black Beans
- Dessert: Gluten-Free Lemon Bars

Day 18

- Breakfast: Chia Seed Pudding

- Lunch: Quinoa and Black Bean Salad
- Snack: Apple Slices with Almond Butter
- Dinner: Roasted Chicken with Sweet Potatoes and Brussels Sprouts
- Dessert: Mango Sticky Rice

Day 19

- Breakfast: Avocado Toast
- Lunch: Mediterranean Chickpea Salad
- Snack: Greek Yogurt with Honey and Walnuts
- Dinner: Spinach and Ricotta Stuffed Shells
- Dessert: Raw Vegan Cheesecake

Day 20

- Breakfast: Greek Yogurt Parfait
- Lunch: Grilled Chicken Salad with Mixed Greens
- Snack: Spiced Chickpea Crunch
- Dinner: Slow Cooker Chicken Stew
- Dessert: Vegan Pumpkin Pie

Day 21

- Breakfast: Oatmeal with Berries and Almonds
- Lunch: Lentil and Vegetable Soup
- Snack: Baked Sweet Potato Chips
- Dinner: Lentil and Vegetable Shepherd's Pie
- Dessert: Vegan Chocolate Truffles

Week 4

Day 22

- Breakfast: Quinoa Breakfast Bowl
- Lunch: Quinoa and Black Bean Salad
- Snack: Caprese Skewers (Cherry Tomatoes, Basil, and Mozzarella)
- Dinner: Herb-Crusted Pork Tenderloin with Steamed Broccoli
- Dessert: Vegan Lemon Poppy Seed Muffins

Day 23

- Breakfast: Blueberry Buckwheat Pancakes
- Lunch: Turkey and Avocado Wrap
- Snack: Avocado and Black Bean Salsa
- Dinner: Baked Cod with Asparagus and Lemon
- Dessert: Vegan Peanut Butter Cups

Day 24

- Breakfast: Spinach and Mushroom Egg White Omelette
- Lunch: Grilled Chicken Salad with Mixed Greens
- Snack: Cucumber and Tomato Salad
- Dinner: Turkey and Vegetable Stir-Fry
- Dessert: Vegan Chocolate Pudding

Day 25

- Breakfast: Smoothie with Spinach and Berries
- Lunch: Lentil and Vegetable Soup

- Snack: Hummus with Veggie Sticks
- Dinner: Stuffed Bell Peppers with Quinoa and Black Beans
- Dessert: Coconut Milk Ice Cream

Day 26

- Breakfast: Chia Seed Pudding
- Lunch: Quinoa and Black Bean Salad
- Snack: Apple Slices with Almond Butter
- Dinner: Roasted Chicken with Sweet Potatoes and Brussels Sprouts
- Dessert: Date and Nut Energy Balls

Day 27

- Breakfast: Avocado Toast
- Lunch: Mediterranean Chickpea Salad
- Snack: Greek Yogurt with Honey and Walnuts
- Dinner: Spinach and Ricotta Stuffed Shells
- Dessert: Dairy-Free Apple Crisp

Day 28

- Breakfast: Greek Yogurt Parfait
- Lunch: Grilled Chicken Salad with Mixed Greens
- Snack: Spiced Chickpea Crunch
- Dinner: Slow Cooker Chicken Stew
- Dessert: Avocado Lime Sorbet

CHAPTER 10: Frequently Asked Questions

Our FAQ section addresses common questions and concerns, providing clear and concise answers to help you feel informed and reassured. We cover a range of topics, from dietary guidelines to exercise recommendations, ensuring you have the information you need.

1. What is congestive heart failure (CHF)?

Congestive heart failure (CHF) is a chronic condition where the heart doesn't pump blood as effectively as it should. This can lead to symptoms such as shortness of breath, fatigue, swollen legs, and fluid retention in the abdomen.

---

2. How does diet impact CHF?

Diet plays a crucial role in managing CHF. A heart-healthy diet can help reduce symptoms, prevent fluid buildup, and improve overall heart function. Key dietary changes include reducing sodium intake, eating balanced meals with plenty of fruits and vegetables, and avoiding foods high in saturated fats and refined sugars.

---

3. What are the key nutrients for heart health?

Important nutrients for heart health include potassium, magnesium, fiber, and omega-3 fatty acids. These nutrients help regulate blood pressure, reduce inflammation, improve blood vessel function, and support overall cardiovascular health.

---

4. Why is sodium reduction important for CHF patients?

High sodium intake can lead to fluid retention, increasing the volume of blood that the heart must pump and exacerbating CHF symptoms. Reducing sodium intake helps manage fluid balance and reduces the workload on the heart.

5. How can I reduce my sodium intake effectively?

To reduce sodium intake, focus on eating fresh, unprocessed foods, such as fruits, vegetables, lean meats, and whole grains. Avoid processed and packaged foods, which often contain high levels of sodium. When cooking, use herbs and spices instead of salt to flavor your meals.

6. What types of exercises are safe for CHF patients?

Gentle, low-impact exercises such as walking, swimming, and stretching are generally safe for CHF patients. It's important to consult with your healthcare provider before starting any new exercise regimen to ensure it is appropriate for your condition.

7. How does physical activity benefit CHF patients?

Regular physical activity strengthens the heart muscle, improves circulation, and enhances overall fitness. Exercise can also help manage weight, reduce stress, and improve energy levels, all of which are beneficial for CHF patients.

8. What are some tips for meal planning and preparation?

Plan your meals ahead of time and make a grocery list to ensure you have healthy ingredients on hand. Prepare meals at home to control ingredients and portion sizes. Batch cooking and freezing meals can save time and help you stick to your dietary goals.

9. How can I manage stress to improve my heart health?

Stress management techniques such as deep breathing exercises, meditation, yoga, and spending time in nature can help reduce stress levels. Regular physical activity and adequate sleep also play a crucial role in managing stress.

10. What should I do if I experience a worsening of my CHF symptoms?

If you experience a worsening of your CHF symptoms, such as increased shortness of breath, swelling, or sudden weight gain, contact your healthcare provider immediately. Early intervention can help prevent complications and improve outcomes.

11. How can I stay motivated to maintain a heart-healthy lifestyle?

Set realistic goals and celebrate your progress, no matter how small. Seek support from family, friends, and healthcare providers. Stay informed about CHF and its management, and remind yourself of the long-term benefits of a heart-healthy lifestyle.

12. Are there any specific foods I should avoid completely?

It's best to avoid foods high in sodium, saturated fats, trans-fats, and refined sugars. This includes processed and packaged foods, fast food, sugary snacks, and beverages, as well as fatty cuts of meat and full-fat dairy products.

13. Can I still enjoy my favorite foods with CHF?

Yes, you can still enjoy your favorite foods by making heart-healthy modifications. For example, you can reduce sodium by using herbs and spices, choose leaner cuts of meat, and use healthier cooking methods such as baking or grilling instead of frying.

14. How can I get my family involved in a heart-healthy lifestyle?

Encourage your family to join you in preparing and eating heart-healthy meals. Share the benefits of a heart-healthy lifestyle with them and involve them in physical activities you can do together. Making it a family effort can provide additional motivation and support.

15. Where can I find more resources and support for managing CHF?

In addition to this cookbook, consult with your healthcare provider for personalized advice and support. Join CHF support groups, either in person or online, to connect with others facing similar challenges. Reliable websites and organizations dedicated to heart health can also provide valuable information and resources.

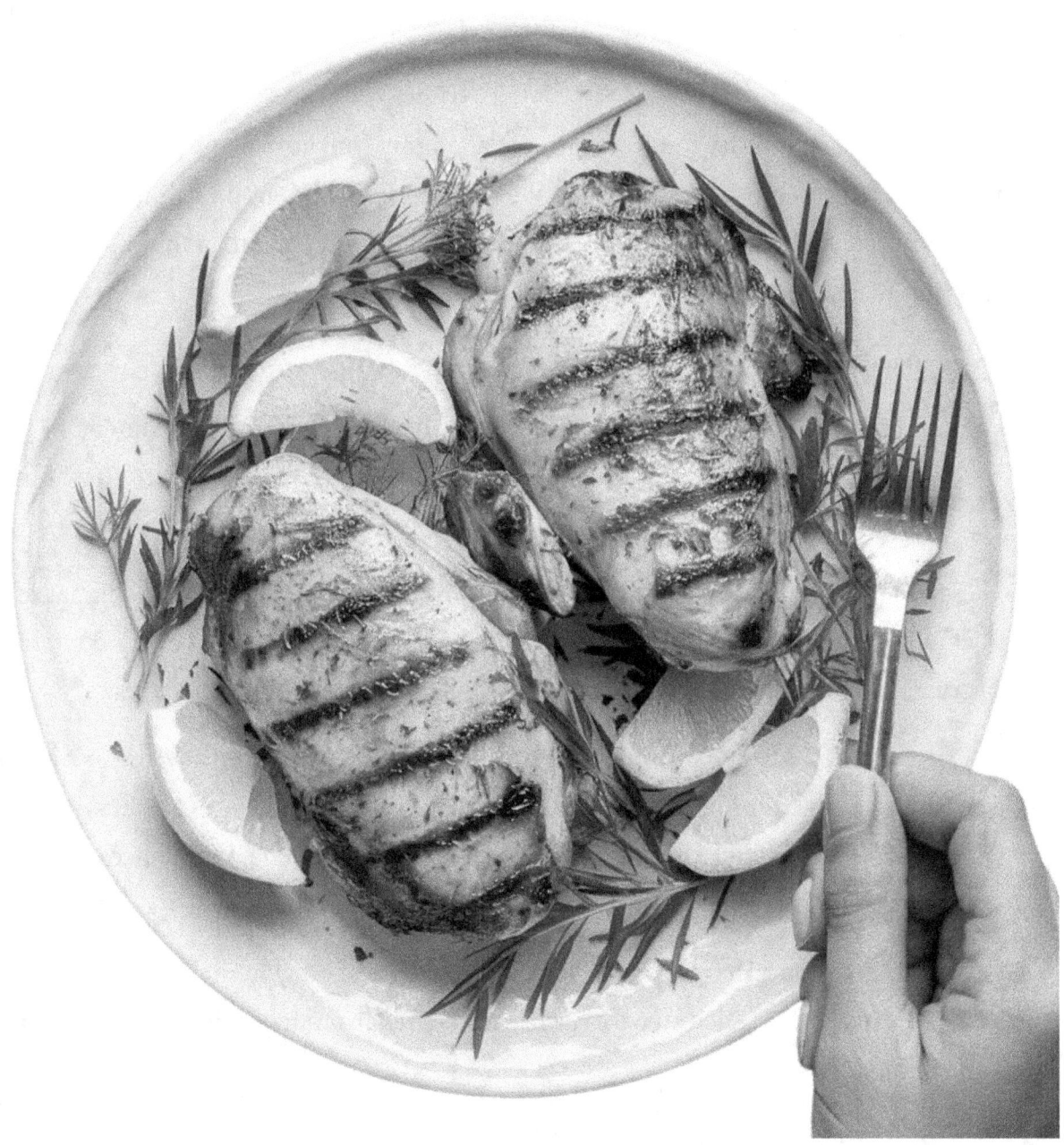

CONCLUSION

Thank you for embarking on this journey with the "Congestive Heart Failure Cookbook." Your commitment to improving your heart health is a significant step towards a better, more vibrant life. As you continue to explore and implement the heart-healthy recipes, meal plans, and lifestyle tips provided in this book, remember that every positive change you make is a victory for your heart and overall well-being.

Living with congestive heart failure can be challenging, but it is also an opportunity to embrace a healthier lifestyle that nourishes your body and uplifts your spirit. The guidance offered in this cookbook is designed to support you in making sustainable changes that will have a lasting impact on your health.

Always keep in mind:

- **You Have the Power:** Every healthy choice you make is a testament to your strength and dedication. You have the power to influence your health through the foods you eat and the lifestyle you lead.

- **Small Steps Lead to Big Changes:** Focus on making small, manageable changes that you can maintain over time. These small steps, when combined, create a powerful path to better health.

- **Community and Support:** You are not alone on this journey. Lean on your family, friends, and healthcare providers for support and encouragement. Share your successes and challenges, and draw strength from the experiences of others who are on the same path.

- **Celebrate Your Progress:** Take pride in the progress you make, no matter how small it may seem. Each step forward is a step towards a healthier heart and a more fulfilling life.

- **Look to the Future:** Your commitment to a heart-healthy lifestyle today paves the way for a healthier tomorrow. Focus on the long-term benefits of the changes you are making. A healthier heart means more energy, better quality of life, and the ability to enjoy more of the moments that matter most.

- **Gratitude and Positivity:** Approach each day with gratitude for the progress you've made and the potential for continued improvement. A positive attitude can make a significant difference in how you experience and manage your health journey. Be kind to yourself, and appreciate the efforts you are making towards a healthier life.

I hope this cookbook serves as a valuable resource and inspiration for you. May the recipes nourish your body, the tips and techniques enhance your lifestyle, and the success stories inspire you to stay committed to your health journey.

Here's to a healthier heart and a brighter future. Your heart deserves the best, and with dedication and the right tools, you can achieve a vibrant, heart-healthy life.

Thank you for trusting the "Congestive Heart Failure Cookbook" as your guide. We wish you all the best on your journey to heart health.

Recap of the Importance of Diet and Lifestyle in Managing CHF

1. Nutritional Guidelines:

- **Balanced Nutrition:** Eating a balanced diet rich in fruits, vegetables, whole grains, lean proteins, and healthy fats is essential for maintaining overall heart health. Proper nutrition helps manage weight, reduce cholesterol levels, and control blood pressure.

- **Sodium Reduction:** High sodium intake can lead to fluid retention, which exacerbates CHF symptoms. Adopting a low-sodium diet helps reduce fluid buildup and decreases the workload on the heart.

- **Key Nutrients:** Certain nutrients, such as potassium, magnesium, fiber, and omega-3 fatty acids, are particularly beneficial for heart health. These nutrients support proper heart function, reduce inflammation, and improve blood vessel health.

- **Hydration:** Proper hydration is essential, but it's important to manage fluid intake to avoid overloading the heart. Discuss with your healthcare provider the right balance for your specific condition.

2. Heart-Healthy Diet:

- **Foods to Include:** Focus on incorporating foods that support heart health, such as leafy greens, berries, nuts, seeds, fatty fish, and legumes. These foods provide essential nutrients and antioxidants that promote cardiovascular health.

- **Foods to Avoid:** Limit or avoid foods high in saturated fats, trans fats, cholesterol, and refined sugars. These can contribute to plaque buildup in arteries and worsen heart conditions.

- **Portion Control:** Managing portion sizes helps prevent overeating and supports weight management, which is crucial for reducing the strain on the heart.

3. Meal Planning and Preparation:

- **Smart Grocery Shopping:** Planning your meals and shopping with a list ensures you have healthy ingredients on hand and reduces the temptation to buy unhealthy options.

- **Cooking at Home:** Preparing meals at home allows you to control the ingredients and cooking methods, ensuring they align with heart-healthy guidelines.

- **Batch Cooking:** Preparing meals in advance can save time and help you stick to your dietary goals, especially on busy days.

4. Lifestyle Changes:

- **Physical Activity:** Regular exercise improves cardiovascular health, strengthens the heart muscle, and enhances overall fitness. Gentle exercises like walking, swimming, and stretching can be beneficial for CHF patients.

- **Stress Management:** Chronic stress can negatively impact heart health. Incorporating relaxation techniques such as deep breathing, meditation, and yoga can help manage stress levels.

- **Adequate Sleep:** Quality sleep is essential for heart health. Establish a regular sleep routine and create a restful environment to promote better sleep.

- **Avoiding Smoking and Limiting Alcohol:** Smoking and excessive alcohol consumption can worsen CHF. Quitting smoking and limiting alcohol intake are critical steps in managing heart health.

5. Support and Education:

- **Healthcare Team:** Work closely with your healthcare providers to monitor your condition, adjust treatments, and receive personalized advice.

- **Education and Resources:** Stay informed about CHF and its management through reliable sources. Use tools like this cookbook to guide your dietary and lifestyle choices.

- **Community and Support Groups:** Connecting with others who are managing CHF can provide emotional support, practical advice, and encouragement.

Conversion Table

Volume Conversions

US Measurement	Metric Measurement
1 teaspoon (tsp)	5 milliliters (ml)
1 tablespoon (tbsp)	15 milliliters (ml)
1 cup	240 milliliters (ml)
1 pint	473 milliliters (ml)
1 quart	946 milliliters (ml)
1 gallon	3.785 liters (L)

Weight Conversions

US Measurement	Metric Measurement
1 ounce (oz)	28 grams (g)
1 pound (lb)	454 grams (g)
1 kilogram (kg)	2.2 pounds (lb)

4. Lifestyle Changes:

- **Physical Activity:** Regular exercise improves cardiovascular health, strengthens the heart muscle, and enhances overall fitness. Gentle exercises like walking, swimming, and stretching can be beneficial for CHF patients.

- **Stress Management:** Chronic stress can negatively impact heart health. Incorporating relaxation techniques such as deep breathing, meditation, and yoga can help manage stress levels.

- **Adequate Sleep:** Quality sleep is essential for heart health. Establish a regular sleep routine and create a restful environment to promote better sleep.

- **Avoiding Smoking and Limiting Alcohol:** Smoking and excessive alcohol consumption can worsen CHF. Quitting smoking and limiting alcohol intake are critical steps in managing heart health.

5. Support and Education:

- **Healthcare Team:** Work closely with your healthcare providers to monitor your condition, adjust treatments, and receive personalized advice.

- **Education and Resources:** Stay informed about CHF and its management through reliable sources. Use tools like this cookbook to guide your dietary and lifestyle choices.

- **Community and Support Groups:** Connecting with others who are managing CHF can provide emotional support, practical advice, and encouragement.

Conversion Table

Volume Conversions

US Measurement	Metric Measurement
1 teaspoon (tsp)	5 milliliters (ml)
1 tablespoon (tbsp)	15 milliliters (ml)
1 cup	240 milliliters (ml)
1 pint	473 milliliters (ml)
1 quart	946 milliliters (ml)
1 gallon	3.785 liters (L)

Weight Conversions

US Measurement	Metric Measurement
1 ounce (oz)	28 grams (g)
1 pound (lb)	454 grams (g)
1 kilogram (kg)	2.2 pounds (lb)

Temperature Conversions

Fahrenheit (°F)	Celsius (°C)
32 °F	0 °C
50 °F	10 °C
75 °F	24 °C
100 °F	38 °C
375 °F	190 °C
425 °F	220 °C

Common Ingredient Conversions

Ingredient	US Measurement	Metric Measurement
All-purpose flour	1 cup	120 grams (g)
Granulated sugar	1 cup	200 grams (g)
Butter	1 cup	227 grams (g)

www.ingramcontent.com/pod-product-compliance
Lightning Source LLC
Chambersburg PA
CBHW082235220526
45479CB00005B/1241